Pranotherapy

the origins of

Polarity Therapy

and

European Neuromuscular Technique

by

Dewanchand Varma
Dr Randolph Stone

including the Dr Stone Notebooks

Pioneers of Manual Medicine Volume I

with additional material and editing

by

Phil Young

MWI Publishing

Published in Great Britain 2011

by
MASTERWORKS INTERNATIONAL
27 Old Gloucester Street London
WC1N 3XX
UK

Email: admin@mwipublishing.com
Web: http://www.mwipublishing.com

ISBN: 978-0-9565803-3-7

Book cover by Mywizarddesign.com

*This book is a historic document and is intended for
use by health care professionals and should not be
regarded as a guide to self-diagnosis or treatment.*

Pranotherapy

the origins of

Polarity Therapy

and

European Neuromuscular Technique

Contents

For Stephanie

in memoriam

May there always be a place for you in Shangri-la

Acknowledgements

I am indebted to Cindy Rawlinson who owns the copyright on the Dr Stone notebooks for permission to publish them. This copyright permission was granted to her by Louise Hilger, Dr Randolph Stone's niece when Louise was the administrator of the Dr Stone Trust.[1] A debt of thanks is owed to Carol Rudd who did the transcription from the original Dr Stone notebooks.

I'm also very grateful to Leon Chaitow ND DO the renowned British trained osteopath for loaning me his copy of 'The Human Machine and its Forces' by Dewanchand Varma some 10 years ago and for filling me in on some historical details of the meeting between Stanley Lief and Dr Randolph Stone. Leon kindly contributed a new foreward to the Varma book and I am also profoundly grateful for all his other writings on the development of European Neuromuscular Technique.

Finally. I wish to pay tribute to my teacher in the art and science of Polarity Therapy Alan Siegel MSc ND and his teacher Pierre Pannetier ND, both of whom passed from this life all too soon.

Preface

In this first decade of the 21st century the very nature of books and the publishing industry is undergoing a profound transformation. This book could quite easily have been created as just an e-book or in the form of a web site on the Internet. However, as a confirmed bibliophile, I believe that there is nothing more rewarding than holding a book in your hands. As Carl Jung said books are not 'just' books, they have a consciousness, and they come to you at the right time. In a similar vein, Jung also said, "Words are animals, alive with a will of their own." So, I hope this book appears in your life at just the right moment to work some kind of transformation that will aid you in your journey in the Healing Arts.

It would be pointless not to utilise the power of modern technology to enhance this work. With that in mind there is a website[1] linked to this book that will have much more related material such as newspaper articles, photographs and audio files. Hopefully, as more material is discovered it too will be added to the web site over time.

It is all too easy for followers of any teacher to re-interpret the teacher's original writings in the light of time and experience, but such a process often does no real service to future generations and can often obscure the original teaching or message, and in some cases completely corrupt it. With this in mind I have done some very mild editing on the Dr Randolph Stone notebooks to make them more easily readable but, in the interests of future research, the original unedited texts are available online for anyone to explore. Also available online are the original recordings which have been transcribed and again mildly edited for this book.

In terms of the print production, the Dewanchand Varma book that we have reproduced in this volume is an extremely close facsimile of the original text. The original book was the same width as this volume but about 1 inch (2.5cms) taller. We have carefully re-typeset the text using a more modern font, the graphics and blank pages are exactly as in the original and the page count is the same. The Dr Randolph Stone notebooks were transcribed from the original notebooks in the early 1980s and we have again re-typeset the transcription and the graphics are placed exactly as in the originals. The notebooks do not follow an exact chronological order as one of the notebooks has material from two different years.

The other material in the book is my own and was added to tie all the material together as well as to give some historical background.

Introduction

This book is the expression of a small part of my exploration of the evolution of a unique approach to manual therapy, developed by Dr Randolph Stone which he called Polarity Therapy. Stone was a pioneer in the integration of vitalistic energy concepts into manual therapy.

My initial training in Polarity Therapy took place in 1984 in San Francisco. During the training I purchased all the books written by Stone. At that time they were in the form of five separate volumes[1] and a number of smaller booklets. I read them all whilst I was training. I very quickly found out why, at various times, Stone had complained that no one read his books after they bought them. They are both dense and, at times, somewhat impenetrable being an eclectic mix of osteopathic and chiropractic technique and reflex zone therapy blended with discussions on Eastern concepts of energy, mysticism, Western Alchemy, New Thought teaching, naturopathic dietary information and more! Stone was indeed a true eclectic.

Eclecticism is a common phenomenon in the field of manual therapy. Most practitioners are multi-disciplinary in their work. Stone's initial training encompassed Osteopathy, Chiropractic and Naturopathy. Later he trained in Neuropathy, the work of Major Bertrand DeJarnette (Bloodless Surgery, S.O.T etc) and Zone Therapy. He explored Naprapathy and Craniopathy and indeed any other system that crossed his path. In the late 1970s, when he was in his eighties, he was exploring magnet therapy.

What distinguishes Stone's work is that he sought to integrate all the disparate approaches to therapy that he had learned in a cohesive way. His answer lay in the original title of his first published book "Energy - The Vital Principle in the Healing Arts," which appeared in 1948. He saw that he could integrate all of the different approaches that he used in his therapeutic work by this single unifying principle of 'energy.' To Stone everything was energy, or as he used to say in his seminars, "Energy is the Keynote" and the effectiveness of any therapeutic approach was directly related to how it influenced the energetic substrate of the body. To Stone, the Soul itself was energy, the Mind was energy and the body was energy too, all vibrating at different frequencies. Another pioneer of manual therapy, an Ayurvedic and yogic practitioner called Dewanchand Varma, who is the other subject of this book, was another of Stone's influences and he too believed in the all pervasiveness of energy. Varma wrote:

> "In the course of long years of research and practice we have sought to discover the law of creation.
> This is our conclusion:
> *Variation of vibration is the cause of creation*
> Vibration is the manifestation and movement of life - it is life itself. The source of all vibration is the universal force known as the Prana,"

Prior to my training in Polarity training I had completed a practitioner training in another energy based bodywork system called Jin Shin Do, but as much as I resonate with Chinese Taoist philosophy, I found Traditional Chinese medicine both complex and contradictory as well as emotionally unsatisfying. Ever since my teenage years I have believed that if something cannot be explained and demonstrated to me in a simple and elegant way then I am unlikely to be able to use it effectively. What I found in Polarity Therapy was a much simpler understanding of energy that resonated more with my Western scientific education, plus a clarity of technique and application. This gave me a deeper emotional satisfaction in the work than anything I had previously experienced. I also realised that it was the only training that I would ever need to do as the system was, in itself, a unique eclectic yet totally integrated blend of a large number of the major approaches to manual therapy that have emerged since the 1880's.

Since the 1970's, Polarity Therapy has been, in my opinion, overly linked with the science of Ayurveda. In part, this is because Stone was an ardent follower of a particular Indian spiritual tradition and because he retired to India permanently in 1973. It is also due to the increasing availability of information on Ayurveda both through books and through Ayurvedic doctors and practitioners coming to live and teach in the West. I have even heard Polarity Therapy called the bodywork of Ayurveda. Numerous Polarity teachers have, over the last three decades, drawn parallels between many different aspects of Polarity Therapy with Ayurvedic models. Personally, I believe this actually misses the core of Polarity Therapy.

History, and how things evolve over time, has always been a fascination for me and lies at the heart of my reasons for publishing this book. Since my early teens I have also enjoyed a free ranging exploration of both Eastern and Western mystical and esoteric teachings. I have a vivid memory from 1969 of, at the age thirteen, talking to my Nan[2] about how modern science was talking about everything as vibration, and being profoundly surprised and intrigued when she said that this was not new and that she had an uncle who was something called a "Theosophist." He had told her the very same thing when she herself was just a young girl in the first decade of the 20th century. This started my reading of Theosophical literature which led me to Rosicrucianism and, over time, on to countless other spiritual and mystical teachings.

You can, perhaps, imagine my curiosity and surprise when on reading Stone's books for the first time, on what I had originally and perhaps naively thought of as just another bodywork system, to find hidden depths in the form of endless references to the Western Alchemical Tradition and the work of Paracelsus as well as Theosophical and Rosicrucian spiritual and mystical teachings.

One of the oddities of Stone's books is that they were all originally self published and as such they were not subject to normal editorial process. Many of the charts he included in his books had no references or citations as to their original sources. He often quotes from specific books but without any indication that they are, in fact, quotes not his own original writings. I saw charts of the 'UPA,' the universal physical atom taken from the theosophical book 'Occult Chemistry,' other charts from the books of Max Heindel on Rosicrucianism and many more uncited references. It was also obvious to me that his language of energy was taken largely from Theosophical sources and writers like Sir Oliver Lodge[3]. It is rather obvious, if you think about it, that the books and information Stone had access to between 1910 and 1950 were not Ayurvedic medical texts but they were the Theosophical versions of the Indian yogic teaching on prana and the chakras brought to the West by authors such as Blavatsky, Besant and Leadbeater[4].

In a short biography of Stone written in January of 1968 by his niece and secretary Louse Hilger, she noted that:

"Dr. Stone never stopped seeking the Spiritual Depths, the Mysteries of Life, as he termed them at that time. He was an avid reader of all the occult, esoteric and hermetic books that he could find,"

"He was a student of Vivekananda's teachings as well as of Swami Rama Tirtha, Yogananda, Krishnamurti, Swedenbourg,

Madam Blavatsky and many others. He was a member of the Philosophical Research Society, having attended Dr. Manly P. Hall's lectures and purchased and read all of his books. He was also a student of Rosicrucianism and Sufism, and was offered the leadership of the Sufis in Chicago at that time."

The influence of the Theosophical teachings on energy and the Indian chakra system is profound but strictly speaking this is not Ayurveda. There is no doubt that after Stone's first trips to India in the 1950's he did indeed incorporate some Ayurvedic concepts into Polarity Therapy, but the system was largely fully formed by 1945 when he began writing his first book. Nor is the Theosophical version of Indian yogic teachings the strongest influence in his work. In fact, and this would require another whole book to explore fully, the Paracelsian influence in his work is very strong and I believe Stone himself had an unconscious identification with Paracelsus or to give him his full name Philippus Aureolus Theophrastus Bombastus von Hohenheim, as Stone's life has many parallels with that of Paracelsus. I have at various times spoken of modern day Polarity Therapists as being "Paracelsian Doctors" in the wake of such figures as Robert Fludd (1574-1637) the great British Alchemist.

The keynote in Polarity Therapy for me is that it is a unique evolution and expression of the Western Mystery traditions applied to manual therapy and as such it is, as Stone might say, "a pearl of great value."

Occasionally, Stone did cite where he got some of his knowledge from and one of those citations is for Pranotherapy which was a system created by the Ayurvedic and yogic practitioner Dewanchand Varma. Stone reproduced all the charts from Varma's book "The Human Machine and its Forces" with some small extra additions in his second book, "The Wireless

13

Anatomy of Man." Stone never met Varma but the book did influence his understandings significantly.

Varma himself was also, as we shall see later, profoundly influential in the genesis of what has been called European Neuromuscular Technique (NMT).

The Evolution of Technique

The development of all forms of manual therapy is subject to profound evolutionary forces. Charles Darwin used the metaphor of a "tree of life" in his book the 'Origin of the Species' to illustrate his ideas about natural selection and the way in which species evolve over time. In most ancient cultures the idea of a tree of life is a universal archetype relating to the interconnectedness of all things.

The work of any founder of a manual therapy system represents, in essence, the trunk of an evolutionary tree for that body of work. The first generation students of the founder often simply follow along in a straight upward path or evolutionary line. However, very quickly as students begin practicing they start to modify the work they learned according to their background knowledge, practical experience and personal bias. So we get evolutionary branches emerging from the main trunk of the tree. These branches often purport to be advances on the original body of work that they emerge from, sometimes being a particular speciality or subset of the work, other times as a simplification of the original work that purports to get to the essential core or perhaps I should say heartwood of the work. These branches often become more successful than the original work and yet in their own way they are often evolutionary dead-ends that eventually die out because they have oversimplified the work or become too specialised. In some cases, you could image that seeds from these successful branches scatter and take root elsewhere ultimately becoming totally separate from the original tree.

To use a different metaphor from our modern computer era, many people will have had the experience of a software update failing to work properly if at all. New versions of a programme or operating system are often not as functional as older versions and many times vital feature sets are deleted. In essence, the founder of any new manual therapy system created and compiled the 'source code' for that approach and the students and teachers who follow afterwards are acting as new programmers who bring their own bias to the development of the code. In some cases they simply apply bug fixes but in many situations interfaces are re-designed, fundamental parameters of the programme are altered and so new code is written and recompiled. In some cases what emerges is indeed an advance on the original and in other cases it is exactly the opposite.

When we learn any technique or skill from a teacher with long therapeutic and teaching experience, what we get is the distillation of all their previous life experience, learning and new discoveries in a nutshell. Yet the nutshell is specific to that particular time in their life and stage of their development. We get the essence of what they believe to be important at that time. Yet this so called 'essence' is often something of a movable feast, as time and experience can dramatically change perceptions and understanding and new discoveries are constantly emerging.

This is a common situation in manual therapy where you find first generation teachers who have all trained with the founder of a system but who experienced the founder's work at a different time and stage in their development. Hence the essence taught to each student is often quite different. After the passing of the founder of the system this more often than not leads to frequent ideological battles over who has the 'true' teaching, the real transmission. I believe the only solution in this situation is to go back to the source material to both re-trace and re-evaluate the evolution of the system. In this way your understanding of the heart of the work is deepened and new insights into the development of the work can emerge.

It is with this in mind that in the first section of this book I offer you a full reprint of the one of the original works of Dewanchand Varma entitled "The Human Machine and its Forces," on his 'Pranotherapy,' as well as a short biography of his life and work.

Dewanchand Varma was deeply instrumental in the creation and evolution of what is now generally referred to as European Neuromuscular Technique (NMT). In the early 1930s osteopath Stanley Lief ND DC studied with Varma and subsequently, Lief together with his cousin Boris Chaitow ND DC, expanded on Varma's work which eventually lead to the creation of European Neuromuscular Technique.

I can only point you to the unique contribution of Leon Chaitow ND DO and Judith DeLany LMT in their work on creating detailed textbooks of NMT and beginning the integration the European and American methods.[1] This integration is truly a unique merging of different evolutionary branches.

Stone's writings on Polarity Therapy, unlike those of Varma, continue to be in print. Stone's books were written between 1945 and 1958.[2] He also wrote newspaper articles for a health column that was published in the Indian newspaper 'The Ambala Tribune,' during 1962 and these, along with a few other small pamphlets, were later consolidated into the book 'Health Building.'

During the last 10 years I have been privileged to read all of Stone's case notes that still exist from 1945 onwards, his other unpublished writings and all of this personal letters exchanged with other practitioners among them such notable figures as Dr Robert Fulford DO. Fulford himself studied with Stone in the early 1960s. I was also able to read all Stone's letters to his successor Pierre Pannetier. I have spent endless hours researching his family background and in 2008 launched a virtual museum on his life.[3]

Audio recordings of Dr Stone's lectures on polarity therapy from 1956 until his last seminars in 1973 have been available for some time. However, most that were in circulation in the 1980s and 1990s were of particularly poor quality, being recorded on inferior equipment and then copied many times. In 2003 I was fortunate enough to have been given a set of audio tapes that were of much higher quality which I spent some months digitally enhancing and which are now available in the form of an audio DVD.[4]

Through Stone's published books it is quite possible to trace the early evolution of his work whereas what his notebooks, which appear at the end of this volume, grant is a unique glimpse into his daily stream of consciousness captured in written form. They were written right at the end of his teaching career. They give a unique insight into his daily life and thought processes and show that he was still exploring and theorising on the nature of life, energy and therapy when he was in his early eighties.

Vitalism

The history of medicine over the last two thousand years has been largely dominated by vitalistic philosophy. In the late 19th century, vitalistic philosophers argued that living organisms are distinguished from inert matter by their possession of a 'life force' that animates them and guides their evolution. The notion of an entelechy or élan vital was widely accepted.

The encyclopaedia Britannica defines vitalism as a "school of scientific thought—the germ of which dates from Aristotle—that explains the nature of life as resulting from a vital force peculiar to living organisms and different from all other forces found outside living things. This force is held to control form and development and to direct the activities of the organism."

The basic theory behind vitalism is that it is not possible to reduce living processes to the mechanical laws of physics and chemistry and that the organism as a whole, is considered greater than the sum of its parts.

In their early development both Osteopathy and Chiropractic were based on vitalistic principles. Andrew Taylor Still, the founder of Osteopathy, constantly talked of the body in terms of mechanics, 'the human machine,' but this foreground focus lay against a background of vitalistic philosophy.

> "As an electrician controls electric currents, so an Osteopath controls life currents and revives suspended forces."
> — Autobiography of A. T. Still

> "I took the position in 1874 that the living blood swarmed with health corpuscles to all parts of the body. Interfere with that current of blood, and you steam down the river of life and land in the ocean of death. That is the discovery. The arteries bring the

blood and wash it with the spirit of life. The living arteries form this world. It fills all space and forms the clouds."
— Autobiography of A. T. Still

"First the material body, second the spiritual being, third a being of mind which is far superior to all vital motions and material forms, whose duty is to wisely manage this great engine of life.
— Philosophy of Osteopathy A. T. Still

The quotes below are from the writings of Dr. J. Martin Littlejohn, PhD MD DO LLD who was First Dean of the College of Osteopathy, Kirksville Missouri, founder of the Chicago College of Osteopathy, and founder of the British School of Osteopathy. The quotes are taken from an article entitled "The Physiological Basis of the Therapeutic Law," and appeared in The Journal of the Science of Osteopathy, Volume 3, Number 4, August, 1902.

"THEORY OF THERAPEUTICS.

The theory of our therapeutics depends on, (1) the vital force, which represents the sum of all vital activities and processes in the body organism, the cosmic energy in man, the energy of understanding and will; and (2) on nutrition, the tissues and organs depending for their vitality and vital activity upon nutritive conditions. Both of these are controlled from the brain. The brain centers represent the higher life, and the different paths from the brain to the body along the nervous system are pathways of distribution in connection with vital force and nutrition. In this we must take account of brain nutrition, in connection with which we get (1) the production of a secretion, the cerebro-spinal fluid, and (2) the generation of nerve energy that passes outside of the brain in the form of waves of vibration."

"THE VITAL FORCE.

In man there is a vital force, so-called because there is no better term. It is not the vital principle or the soul or the subjective mind. It is the vital force, or that force which originates and remains in the body as the result of the union of spirit or simple substance with matter. It is the objective mind of the psychologist.

The principle of this vital force is *the power of fluxion or of vibration*, which, as in the physical forces, can permeate the substance without affecting or modifying its substance. There are thus three planes, the pure *material*, the pure *spirit* or psychic, and the plane which originates in connection with the union of these other two, the vital *force* plane."

D.D. Palmer, the Founder of Chiropractic, work was deeply rooted in vitalism. In 1914 he wrote:

"The science of chiropractic is in no way related to the science of machinery. Its phenomena are dependent upon vital force, not that of dynamics.

The structure of the body is defined under that of anatomy, not metalography — a treatise on metals.

Bodily functions depend upon vital force, not dynamics. The existence of metals, whether in the form of machinery or that of ore, depends upon certain inanimate qualities, whereas the existence of animals depends upon functions.

Vital philosophy and mechanical philosophy are not correlated, they are radically and entirely different.

The laws which govern the existence of animated beings and that of animated objects differ.

Chiropractic science is being enlarged and urged on to a higher development by the demands of the art of vertebral adjusting. Why not make use of the knowledge which composes the science?

21

In chiropractic, you should discriminate between science and art. Science depends upon principles, and art upon practice.

The theories of chiropractic become demonstrated facts, the practice an art.

Biology and chiropractic include vital phenomena in contradistinction to physical facts; those functions, energies and acts that depend upon life, as manifested by contrast to those which exist without intelligence."

The early 1920s saw materialism and reductionist philosophy take a stronger and more pervasive hold and largely displaced vitalism as a valid conceptualisation of living processes in the practice of medicine, eventually giving rise to "modern evidence based scientific medicine." This influence of materialism in medicine has been profound and has influenced all its branches. Manual medicine has not been immune. By the late 1930s vitalism began to lose any influence in manual therapies and continues to do so to this day. Even a cursory review of modern literature on manual therapies such as Osteopathy, Chiropractic, massage, Neuromuscular Technique and myofascial work shows that the field is dominated by a materialistic philosophy of life.

Dr Randolph Stone DO DC ND, the founder of Polarity Therapy and one of the major figures featured in this book trained in an early, more vitalistic approach to manual therapy (1912-1916). Uniquely for the time, Stone maintained and deepened a vitalistic orientation in his work contrary to the modern trend but by the 1950s he found himself ostracised by his osteopathic peers as the osteopathic journals in the USA refused to accept adverts for his courses.[1] This situation was mostly due to his continuing linkage of Osteopathy with a vital life force or life energy, a stance that was in complete opposition to the continuing invasion of materialistic philosophy into manual therapy.

In spite of vitalism now being largely discounted by mainstream science, it is the foundation of many types of alternative medicine such as acupuncture and oriental bodywork and some of the Western evolutions of manual therapy. One of the biggest mistakes that has taken place in the Healing Arts since the early 1920s and the rise of materialism, has been the quest to explain the 'life force, prana or chi' in terms that are acceptable to Western reductionist physics. From the 1880s, beginning with the rise of the Theosophical movement, which was itself largely instrumental in bringing Indian yogic models of reality to the West by introducing the concepts of prana and the chakras, there has been an attempt to tie these vitalistic concepts into western physiological models. The chakras were, in the early days of the last century, often related either to various nerve plexus in the body or to certain endocrine glands and the movement of the prana through the body linked to the function of the nervous system.

One of the challenges with vitalism in relation to manual therapy is the fact that physical manipulation on the bones, muscles, ligaments, tendons and skin of the physical body appears to release the flow of life force. This inevitably gives rise to the idea that somehow the life force is 'in' the physical body and has led to an ongoing search for the location of this life energy in the physical body. The work of Stone in Polarity Therapy illustrates this difficulty beautifully. In his early writings in the 1940s, he speaks of the bulk of the prana in circulation in the body as being carried by the blood stream and is related to the Osteopathic concept of the 'artery rules.' By the 1960s, he is talking about the energy as being in the cerebrospinal fluid and then by the 1970s

23

the energy has become a plasma gas carried in the connective tissue.

Another aspect of this problem is the use of science to give credibility to the particular work in question. However, rather than being a real scientific explanation, it is what I call, 'Sunday supplement science.' In the field of journalism there are reporters who specialise in science and scientific discoveries. They have a particular talent for explaining complex scientific theories in simple layman's terms. They often write articles on new discoveries in physics, chemistry or medicine that then appear in the glossy Sunday newspaper supplements.

It is important to remember that very few pioneers in the field of manual therapy are properly trained in physics and yet physics is the field where 'energy' is still explored, albeit energy that is measurable within the electromagnetic spectrum. So when any pioneer sees a new scientific discovery in the Sunday newspapers it is truly tempting to use it to validate their teaching. However, by the time the 'scientific explanation' has gone through secondary and even tertiary reinterpretations it is little more than science as a metaphor not a reality.

Stone often used, this so-called, Sunday supplement science, to elaborate and to some degree justify his work. Even the name of Polarity Therapy itself is to some degree a scientific metaphor. As early as 1916 he had begun using scientific metaphor to explain his discoveries. One early example is the creation of what he called, the 'North Pole stretch,' clearly beginning to view the body as having some kind of electromagnetic structure. Scientific discoveries since that time, utilising Superconducting Quantum Interference Devices (SQUID), have indeed mapped out a bio-magnetic structure to the human body but it is not exactly the same as Stone's formulations or theorisation. He was also familiar with such terms as uni-polar and bi-polar and used them in relation to his teaching. Originally, he came across these terms in his early studies of zone therapy, the precursor to modern reflexology. Zone therapy is yet another early example of scientific metaphor being used to give credibility to a therapy.

This use of scientific metaphor is also often done for marketing purposes. There is a general feeling that if you can explain something in terms of science then it is generally much more acceptable and more powerful regardless of its accuracy. This belief largely arises from the all pervasive role that science plays in the field of education and in the many applications of scientific discoveries in our everyday lives in the form of new media and communication systems. Quantum Touch[2] which is a popular modern, and in my opinion, simplified offshoot of Polarity Therapy clearly uses this aspect of the power of our belief in science. Many other healing systems also invoke what you might call the 'quantum gods.'

The problem with this use of scientific metaphor is that it muddies the waters in terms of developing a deep understanding of the true nature of the work.

The process of looking for the deeper truly scientific foundations of many of the healing arts culminated in the 1990s with the publication of the book, *Energy Medicine the Scientific Evidence* by James Oschman.[3] I found the book an admirable piece of work in many ways but I was also profoundly disappointed by it. In no way did it really speak to my experiences as a practitioner of an energy healing approach that is profoundly embedded in the vitalistic tradition. The book essentially fell into the same trap of trying to explain 'life energy' in terms of a multitude of electromagnetic processes. Although to some extent the book focused on the effects rather than the energy itself.

Whilst it may be possible to talk about the effects of energy work in terms of many different scientific processes it is my contention that the 'energy' that is spoken about in the practice of vitalistic healing arts is in no way related to the processes that can be described by modern Western physics. This was highlighted in a delightfully succinct way by Dr Harold J. Morowitz Ph.D professor of molecular biophysics at Yale university who, upon attending a lecture on Massage Therapy, found himself incensed by the lecturers use of the term 'energy' because as Morowitz pointed out later, it clearly violated or did not obey either the first or second law of thermodynamics. He was to write later in an essay called "Whose Energy?"

"Particularly upsetting talk/was the fact that the bioenergetic notions of the speaker were close enough to the ideas of normal life science to imply that they were the same, even though the masseurs statements were unconstrained by the most elementary laws of physics. This freewheeling sport, using the recovery of science, is a characteristic of many schools ranging from astrology to branches of psychiatry at hand, I believe, universally leads to a kind of mental fogginess."
— Harold J. Morowitz 1979 [4]

Moshe Feldenkrais the creator of the Feldenkrais method of neurological re-education was often told by students, and by his client's, that he had healing hands but he was never happy with this idea.

"I have some difficulty in explaining to my followers that I am not a therapist and my touching has no therapeutic or healing value, though people improve through it. I think that what happens to them is learning, but few agree with this."
— Introduction - the Elusive Obvious

"How can such changes in mood and attitude be brought about by just touching, however cleverly, another person's body? My pupils try to convince me that I possess the healing touch. I have taught students to do what I do in Israel, the United States, and elsewhere, so that they all now have "healing hands". They were not specially chosen, but they were selected for their academic education and their wish and capacity to learn."

— Introduction - The Elusive Obvious

As a physicist who worked in the Joliot-Curie laboratory in Paris in the early 1930s he was generally not happy with the concept of vitalistic life energy. He would often say when questioned about it by his students, "Show it to me, show me this energy."

Yet towards the end of his teaching career he said that you could hold your hand just above a damaged knee and then imagine that the hand was like a sun radiating light on it and that this would make the knee function more efficiently as well as reduce pain. Some of the students protested that he was doing energy healing work to which he simply shrugged and replied, "I don't know what it is but it seems to work." [5]

The real difficulty lies in the actual definition of, or perhaps I should say perception of, life energy. To illustrate a part of the problem, I remember once working on a Feldenkrais practitioner's painful spine at a dinner table doing some Polarity Therapy energy work. After a few minutes he said, "What are doing." I replied "Energy work." He responded by saying that it felt like good Feldenkrais functional integration work to him!

The reality, I believe, is that the energy that is used in all 'energy healing work' is not something that exists within the electromagnetic spectrum. It may well have an impact upon electromagnetic energies and physical structures within the body but it does not itself exist within the physical plane of existence. At this stage I have to apologise to readers who have immediately

27

switched off at the introduction of the idea of different "planes of existence" which is, itself, an old vitalistic terminology. It is a terminology very familiar to any student of Stone's writings. However, it is difficult concept to grasp. Dion Fortune, a Western occultist, was quite eloquent in discussing the concept:

> "We use the word "plane" for these different aspects of existence because it is a term that has been established by usage, but it is in many ways an unfortunate term and leads to misapprehension because it teaches us to think of different types of existence as lying one above the other like the layers of the atmosphere, whereas the different"planes" are really but different modes of manifestation of force. Each "keeps itself to itself" in that it only acts and reacts among its own type of existence, and is oblivious of all other types save when translations are made up and down the planes by the modes we have described."[6]

One of Stone's basic formulations was that "pain is blocked energy"and elsewhere he often commented that "pain is in the astral plane." Another quote from Dion Fortune is illuminating.

> "The astral plane is a plane of 'force' and the physical plane is a plane of 'form.' That gives you the clue to a great deal if you think out its implications. Do you realize that there is no force on the physical plane and no form on the astral?"[7]

To some this might seem little more than potentially disputatious philosophy and so it might be better to simply say that this life energy is 'metaphysical' but perhaps that just takes us deeper into a semantic quicksand. Actually, I suspect it is more appropriate that, in place of the phrase "life energy," that we could use another word or concept entirely and I suggest that the word and concept we could use instead would be 'consciousness.'

All good healers whether they are allopathic medical doctors or practitioners of the most obscure variation of bodywork or energetic healing use their consciousness in specific ways. It is really the use of specific modes or perhaps qualities of consciousness that is intrinsic to energy work.

One of the major problems facing any 'scientific' research into vitalistic processes is that. if it is a function of consciousness or even consciousness itself, it is almost impossible to maintain the appropriate level of consciousness needed to demonstrate this life force energy in laboratory conditions. Russian philosopher P. D. Ouspensky was perhaps the first point out this difficulty.[8]

Any subject in a stringent research study may be able to hold the appropriate state of consciousness for perhaps only a few minutes at a time at best, out of the many hours required to have a process be properly repeatable and measurable. One of the basic facts of human consciousness is that we get bored easily and that when we are under pressure doubts creep in to our consciousness no matter how certain we may be in our healing abilities. If this is an accurate formulation then normal scientific evidence based research on life energy and healing is ultimately doomed because the results are going to be intrinsically variable.

The two pioneers in the history of manual therapy who appear in this book are both guilty, in my opinion, of the error of trying to make this "pranic life energy" and its application in healing, both understandable and acceptable to the modern Western scientific mindset. Varma, as you will see later when you read his book, related the prana to electromagnetic and nerve currents in the body. Stone, originally used electromagnetic terminology extensively when talking about the life energy and in his final years related the life energy to "plasma gas."

From 1970 until he retired from teaching in 1973 Stone often referred to the work of Hannes Alfvén who won the Nobel Prize for Physics 1970 'for fundamental work and discoveries in magnetohydro-dynamics with fruitful applications in different parts of plasma physics.'

In a seminar given in August 1972 Stone said:

"I put this in my books in such a simple manner linking the subtle with the gross, of course I did not have this advanced work of what I am telling you now because they had not given the Nobel prize yet. I could not have told you what it is all about. I could only tell you that the energy did flow and you said "What is it (this energy)? and now because we call it the plasma gas...it 'is' something but before that you called it magnetism, well that was hocus pocus, of course, and that's why I want to dissociate magnetism from this gas because the gas is a primary and magnetism is a radiation like the magnets from iron and so on and that has its own field and it isn't near as effective as the plasma gas."

The decision to talk about the energy in terms of plasma gas was again clearly an attempt by Stone to persuade students in the early 1970s of the 'reality' of energy. It appeared he was trying to convince them that the information he was sharing with them was 'scientifically valid.' In actual fact, this sort of 'proof' probably wasn't necessary as, by this time, most of the alternatively minded students attending Stone's seminars were already sold on the basic concept of energy. This was quite a contrast to the situation Stone faced in his earlier seminars in the 1950's which were given mostly to osteopaths and chiropractors who clearly did not 'get' any form of vitalistic concept and in the seminars could not wait to get on to the 'practical' hands on manipulations.

The acceptance of 'the life force or life energy' as something real, valid and tangible was pervasive throughout all the active counter culture movements of the 1970s such as the Human

Potential movement as well as in the burgeoning field of Alternative Medicine.

Later in the same 1972 seminar Stone said:

> *"I want you to see these energies in space, so when I show you some of this space action I give you magnets to pull you will see the actual force and you will know we are dealing with energy then having established that and found out why it works then you see it IS something. If you don't know why and you can't select it and... well its difficult"*

Stone's concern here seems to be with the essential aspect of *belief* when working with the life energy which links back to our earlier discussion of energy as being fundamentally related to consciousness.

In a sense it is a tribute to the dominance of the modern scientific world view which pervades our whole educational system that nearly all creators and teachers of healing systems, based upon vitalistic philosophies, feel that they have to resort to trying to justify their work in the scientific language of the day. I am certain, that in their own minds, both Stone and Varma knew that their work was actually deeply rooted in the workings of, or perhaps I should even say mysteries of, human consciousness and its application to healing.

> "So long as one knows nothing of a psychic existence, it is projected if it appears at all.
>
> Thus the first knowledge of the laws and rules of the psyche was found in the stars, and further knowledge in unknown matter...
>
> The really important psychic elements cannot be measured with the ruler, or the balance, or the test-tube, or the microscope."
> (Carl Jung - Collected Works 13 The Spirit Mercurius para.148)

Dewanchand Varma
A Brief Biography

Professor Dewanchand Varma, an Ayurveda practitioner and yogi appeared in Paris sometime around 1913. He was, according to newspaper reports of the time, originally a dealer in fine pearls. He was a prolific author with some five titles to his name, some being published in both English and French. In the 1920s and 30s he had a clinic at 32 Rue Spontini in Paris and treated a huge variety of patients, many being extremely ill with diseases such as tuberculosis and congestive heart failure. Whilst living in Paris he published a regular bi-monthly journal on health matters and held weekly meetings of 'The League of Health' at his studio.

His success was such that in the 1927 and again in 1933[1] he attracted the unwelcome attention of the French medical authorities who brought various legal actions against him because he was not medically qualified in France nor worked under the prescription of a French medical doctor.

He vigorously denied these charges but the first case resulted in him receiving a fine and the latter case resulted in a one month custodial sentence. Many of his patents came to court to testify in his defence. It seems highly likely that in the 1920s he was initially unaware of the French legal position for lay practitioners. It is interesting to note that the French court did not make any claim that his methods, which included what he called "pranotherapy" and magnetic treatment as well as yoga and hydrotherapy, were ineffective just that he was not following the legal requirements under which a lay practitioner could give a 'medical' treatment.

From the newspaper articles of the time it seems that, in bringing the civil action, there was a definite element of jealousy on the part of the Parisian medical establishment in that Varma was so successful that the local doctors were losing out financially as so many potential patients went to him to receive his work.

Varma relocated from France to England sometime before the Nazi occupation of Paris and took up residence at 82 Park Mansions in Knightsbridge in London from 1941 through to 1946. During and immediately after the second world war Varma continued his healing work as shown by various magazine and newspaper articles from 1946.[2] According to the articles of the time he was eighty years old in 1946. There are no records of him after 1946.

Varma was also a prolific inventor. Apart from his "pranograph" an apparatus for visually showing energetic disturbances, between the years 1941 - 1946 Varma took out patents on an improved silencer for internal combustion engines, improvements in or relating to air intake devices for carburettors, a seat cushion specially designed to reduce pressure on vital pelvic structures. The scope of his patents is such that he appears to have gained a good degree of engineering knowledge somewhere in his background. He also patented finger grip exercise equipment.[3] The first paragraphs of the patent document for this device reproduced below are interesting in that it shows his interest was very much in rehabilitation, an obvious extension of his therapeutic work and something of significant interest to any bodyworker in terms of the continued healthy functioning of their own hands.

> "I, Dewanchand Varma, a British Subject, of 82, Park Mansions, Knightsbridge, London, S.W.1, do hereby declare the nature of this invention to be as follows :—

This invention relates to finger grips for physical exercises whereby contracted muscles and nerves can be restored to their normal relaxed condition, thereby assisting in regularising the circulation of the blood and lymph.

Since such exercises are directed to muscular relaxation, that is to say gentle and progressive outward extension as opposed to a muscular load or inward contraction such as takes place with strengthening apparatus involving the extension of springs and the like, it is important to reduce to a minimum any tendency for the user to clutch the finger grip in the palm and thereby contract the hand muscles and those of the arm associated therewith."

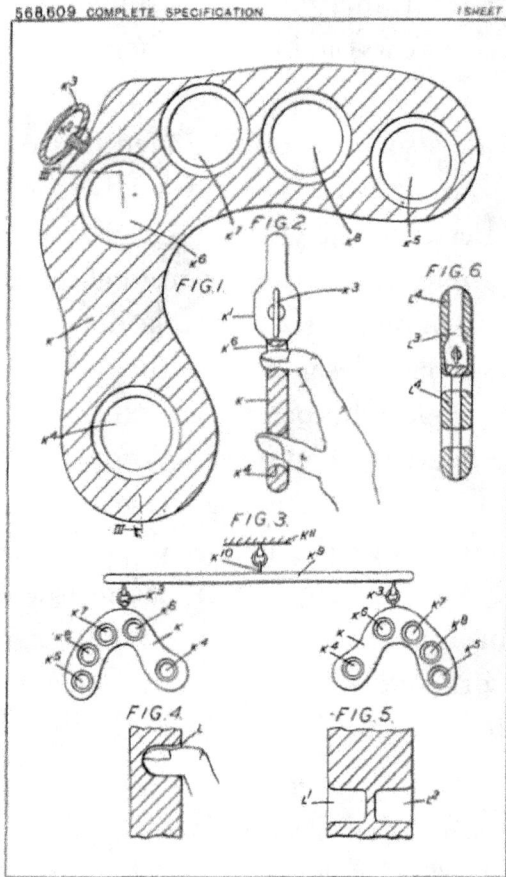

568,609 COMPLETE SPECIFICATION   1 SHEET

FIG. 2.
FIG. 1.
FIG. 6.
FIG. 3.
FIG. 4.
FIG. 5.

Malby & Sons. Photo-Litho

Pranotherapy

Varma primarily practiced what he called Pranotherapy, a form of soft tissue manipulation designed to release palpable obstructions in the physical body. He would apply variable pressure to the muscular tissues of the body. His technique involved first separating the skin from the underlying tissue and then a gentle separation of the muscle fibres using both horizontal and vertical strokes.

Varma described ways in which the prana or electro-magnetic currents of the body, derived from the atmosphere, could become obstructed giving rise to adhesions and hardening of the muscle fibres such that the pranic or nerve currents could not flow through them.

Varma maintained that these blockages were caused by trauma, infection and physiological dysfunction, and that soft tissue changed in relation to mental, emotional problems and changes in the chakras. He wrote extensively on his work in both French and English with such titles as 'The Key to Health,' 'The Education of the Nervous System' and the title reproduced in this volume 'The Human Machine and its Forces.'

Polarity Therapy and NMT

Varma was influential both in the development of Polarity Therapy and Neuromuscular Technique.

Dr Randolph Stone had come to a similar understanding of the role of energetic disturbances when he founded his method of natural healing which he called Polarity Therapy. When Stone came across Varma's work through his writings he was sufficiently impressed with the concepts and methodology that he incorporated all of the charts from Varma's book on Pranotherapy in to his second book, 'The Wireless Anatomy of Man' and added some extra material to the charts that related to the anatomy of the muscle fibres and the connective tissues. Dr Stone was still referring to Varma's work as late as 1973 in his final year of teaching before retiring to India.

Neuromuscular Technique

Stanley Lief, whom we met briefly in the chapter on the evolution of technique was born in Latvia in 1890. He later trained as an osteopath and naturopath in America at Bernarr McFadden's college before relocating to the United Kingdom. Lief later became the founder of British College of Osteopathic Medicine (formerly - The British College of Naturopathy and Osteopathy). He was well known in England for his therapeutic work and in 1926 he founded the renowned health resort at Champneys near Tring, Buckinghamshire and maintained a private practice in London. Lief heard of Varma's work in Paris and went there to receive sessions from him in the early 1930s and later persuaded Varma to come to his clinic in Park Lane to both teach and give sessions. Together with his cousin Boris Chaitow ND DC, Lief incorporated much of what they learned into a system of manual therapy that Lief later called Neuromuscular Technique. The soft tissue manipulations taught by Varma were expanded upon by Lief and Chaitow to include various new techniques over time, a process continued to this day (2011) by Boris Chaitow's nephew Leon Chaitow ND DO. Leon Chaitow speaks more to the origins of Neuromuscular Technique in his foreward to Varma's book "The Human Machine and its Forces" that follows this section.

Lief and Stone both recognised that osseous corrections alone were not enough and that soft tissue manipulation is an important part of manual therapy. Whilst Lief continued to develop the physical soft tissue aspects in the development of Neuromuscular Technique Stone continued to evolve the energetic approach alongside the physical work. In the later chapter on the connective tissue we will explore a meeting that took place between Lief and Stone in which they discussed Varma's work. It is unclear to what degree, if any, that Lief continued to use the energetic model as taught by Varma in his own practice but the quote below is intriguing.

> "Lief also possessed a remarkable instinctive understanding of the human body. As one admirer noted, His powers of diagnosis were extraordinary and his skilled manipulation uncanny in its accuracy. That he possessed healing powers and could transmit healing energy by touch I have no doubt."
>
> Elliot Gorst, 1963. "Stanley Lief: More Personal Tributes."
> Health for All 37:670

Foreword to New Edition

"The Human Machine and its Forces"

by Leon Chaitow ND DO

These notes represent a personal perspective based on the ways in which the ideas and the work of Dr Dewanchand Varma became a part of my clinical approach to health management.

When I was studying osteopathy and naturopathy in London in the late 1950s I was taught Neuromuscular Technique (NMT) as part of our soft-tissue assessment and treatment course. The version of NMT that I learned had been developed in the 1930s by my father's cousin, Stanley Lief ND DC, assisted by his cousin, my uncle Boris Chaitow ND DC.

Lief told us that he had modified a technique, taught to him by a Dr Varma, an Ayurvedic physician working in Paris in the late 1920s, early 1930s. It may be of interest to know that among the people in contact with Varma at that time (according to Lief) was Ida Rolf – although whether she incorporated any of Varma's work into hers is not known. Lief persuaded Dr.Varma to come to London, where he worked in Lief's practice (144 Park Lane), for some years, during which time Varma's book was published by Lief's imprint "Health for All Publications."

Varma believed that the manual treatment method he practiced (he called it "Prana-therapy") and which he taught to Lief, was capable of identifying and treating local areas of obstruction to the free flow of energy, using skilful, intelligent, finger or thumb strokes, and applied pressure.

Lief found the subtle techniques employed by Varma gentle and efficient – essentially involving as they did a 'meeting and

39

matching' of tissue tension, in order to identify – and where necessary modify – freedom, or lack of freedom of motion within these tissues.

Lief used his modifications of Varma's approach – which he called NMT - to assess and treat soft-tissue dysfunction, preparing joints for mobilisation or manipulation. And this is why we were taught NMT in our training at the then British College of Naturopathy and Osteopathy (now renamed as the British College of Osteopathic Medicine).

By the time I was being trained the early work of Janet Travell MD was available and we began to speak of trigger points as one of our targets in NMT assessment and treatment. Simultaneously – in the late 1950s/early 1960s the work of Raymond Nimmo DC was becoming more widely known. Nimmo had worked in parallel with Travell (and subsequently another major researcher into myofascial pain, David Simons MD) in describing localised soft tissue changes that could generate local and distant pain – myofascial trigger points. When Nimmo came to the UK to teach briefly in the early 1960s, I was privileged to attend his classes, and found that his terminology was different from that of Travell, as were his treatment methods (which he called Receptor Tonus Technique) – but that they could usefully be harmonised clinically with Lief's methods. This is what has happened, as NMT has continued to evolve in both the UK and USA. (Chaitow & DeLany 2011)

Lief's (European) modified version of Varma's approaches, NMT, became a superbly effective soft tissue assessment and treatment protocol. The delicacy of the finger or thumb strokes allowing for extremely fine work to be performed – involving intelligent contacts that do not overwhelm restrictions, but insinuate ('melting') their way into them, teasing and releasing, rather than aggressively forcing change – and it is this degree of subtlety that Lief learned almost entirely from Varma.

In the USA Neuromuscular Therapy evolved in a direction that was far more focused on myofascial pain in general (influenced by Travell, Simons and Nimmo), and trigger points in particular. The modalities used in American NMT comprise soft tissue methods developed by practitioners of massage therapy, osteopathy, chiropractic, physical therapy, manual medicine, naturopathic medicine, and others. (Chaitow & Delany 2011)

Varma's visionary perspective- connective tissue connections

In his book 'The Human Machine and Its Forces' Dr. Dewanchand Varma says:

> 'We have discovered that the circulation of the nervous currents, slows down occasionally because of the obstruction caused by adhesions; the muscular fibres harden and the nervous currents can no longer pass through them. We have demonstrated effective and positive methods designed to restore nervous equilibrium which promotes the healthy circulation of blood, so that new tissues begin to be built up again'

In these words Varma seems to be discussing obstructions in the connective tissue – something that is recognised today as fascia research expands exponentially.

Lief had become interested in fascia/connective tissue many years earlier than his introduction to Varma, via the work of a Scottish physician, Dr Andrea Rabagliati (1843-1930).

In 1916 Rabagliati had published a book "Initis – nutrition and exercise" that advanced the theory that connective tissue congestion played a significant part in the etiology of dysfunction and disease. Dr. Varma maintained that it was possible, using what he termed 'pranatherapy', to both palpate and normalise soft tissue restrictions that interfered with what he envisioned as the normal flow of energy ("prana") around the body.

Osteopathic practitioner and educator, Tom Dummer DO, who had studied NMT with Lief in the 1950s, has noted (in an unpublished monograph, dated 1991)):

"Lief noticed the similarity between the theories and techniques of Dr Varma and Dr Rabagliatti and realized that they were virtually complementary to each other. It was from the synthesis of the two that neuromuscular technique eventually evolved."

Writing in the 1960s, Brian Youngs ND DO – who had studied and worked with Stanley Lief, observed as follows:

"Connective tissue ......was largely ignored until recently, but has now been made the subject of close study in regard to its structure and functions. The ubiquity of connective tissue caused Rabagliatti to compare it to the ether - as the medium for, as he termed it, 'the zoodynamic life force.' Through the connective tissues' planes run the trunks and plexuses of veins, arteries, nerves, and lymphatics. Connective tissue is the support for the structural and, therefore, functional relationships of these systems...... and as (NMT) operates primarily on connective tissue it will usually be concentrated at those areas where such tissue is most dense, e.g. muscular origins and insertions, especially the broad aponeurotic insertions .....connective tissue is, after all, ubiquitous"

This brings us right up to date, where research at major institutions is highlighting the role of fascia in both function and dysfunction, much of it echoing the work of Rabagliatti, Varma and Lief.

For example, in relation to function McCombe (2001) has observed:

- "Fascia forms a gliding interface with underlying muscle [allowing] free excursion of the muscle under the relatively immobile skin. A plane of potential movement exists in the form of the areolar tissue layer, [apparently] lined with a lubricant, hyaluronic acid."

While in regard to dysfunction:

- "When fascia is excessively mechanically stressed, inflamed or immobile, collagen and matrix deposition becomes disorganized, resulting in fibrosis and adhesions – fascial thickening' Langevin et al 2008, 2009))
- "Densification occurs, involving distortion of myofascial relationships, altering muscle balance and proprioception" (Stecco et al 2009)
- "Binding occurs among layers, that should stretch, glide and/or shift on each other, potentially impairing motor function" (Fourie 2009)
- Chronic tissue loading occurs, forming 'global soft tissue holding patterns' (Myers 2009)

All of these quotes could have come from Varma – and so I will requote his observation, which was 80 years ahead of this current research – even though the terminology belongs to a time long gone:

'We have discovered that the circulation of the nervous currents, slows down occasionally because of the obstruction caused by adhesions; the muscular fibres harden and the nervous currents can no longer pass through them. We have demonstrated effective and positive methods designed to restore nervous equilibrium which promotes the healthy circulation of blood, so that new tissues begin to be built up again'

Research

As far as NMT's efficacy - research validation is slowly appearing– for example:

- Nagrale and colleagues (2010) demonstrated the efficacy of NMT methods that were incorporated into a focused trigger point protocol - Integrated Neuromuscular Inhibition Technique – INIT (Chaitow 1994).

- Spanish researchers (Ibáñez-García J et al 2009) showed that NMT (Lief's method) and Strain/counterstrain were equally effective in the management of latent trigger points in the masseter muscle.

And of course - in addition to Varma's influence on NMT - there is also his connection with Polarity Therapy – about which I know too little to comment, but which appears to have been just as profound.

There also remains a tantalising possibility that Varma may have influenced the work and thinking of Ida Rolf.

We owe Dr Varma our thanks, and the republication of his book is a fitting tribute.

Leon Chaitow ND DO
Corfu, Greece 2011
www.leonchaitow.com

References

Chaitow L Delany J 2011 Clinical Applications of Neuromuscular Techniques. Volume 2: Lower Body (2nd edition). ChurchillLivingstone, Edinburgh

Chaitow L 1994 Integrated Neuromuscular Inhibition Technique British Jnl of Osteopathy 13:17-20

Dummer T 1991 (unpublished) The Lief Neuromuscular Technique. Maidstone, Kent.

Fourie W 2009 IN: Fascial Research II: Basic Science and Implications for Conventional and Complementary Health Care Munich: Elsevier Gmbh

Ibáñez-García J et al 2009 Changes in masseter muscle trigger points following strain-counterstrain or neuro-muscular technique JBMT 13(1): 2-10

Langevin H 2008.. In: Audette, Bailey (Eds.) Integrative Pain Medicine. Humana

Langevin H 2009 Fascial Research II: Basic Science and Implications for Conventional and Complementary Health Care Munich: Elsevier GmbH

McCombe D et al 2001 Jnl. Hand Surgery 26B:2: 89-97

Myers T 2009 Anatomy Trains, 2nd edition Edinburgh: Churchill Livingstone

Nagrale et al 2010 Efficacy of an integrated neuromuscular inhibition technique on upper trapezius trigger points in subjects with non-specific neck pain. Jnl Manual & Manipulative Therapy 18(1):37-43

Rabagliatti A 1930, 2nd Edition. Original 1916) Initis Or Nutrition and Exercises C. W. Daniel Company, London,

Stecco L Stecco C 2009 Fascial Manipulation: Practical Part. Piccin Italy

Youngs B. 1963 The physiological background of neuromuscular technique. Br Naturopathic Jnl & Osteopathic Rev. 5:176–178

REPRODUCTION OF

THE
HUMAN MACHINE
AND ITS FORCES

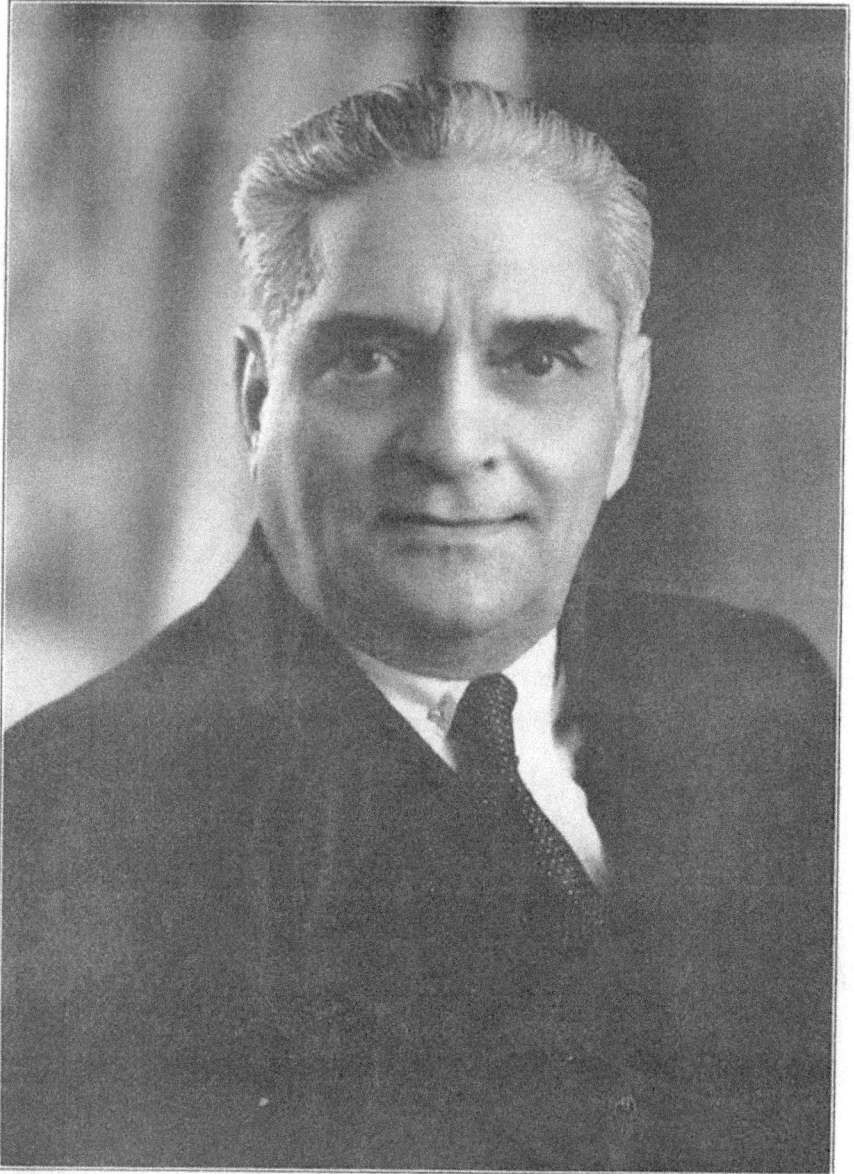

The Author

THE
HUMAN MACHINE
AND ITS FORCES

By

DEWANCHAND VARMA

Pioneer of Pranotherapy

LONDON:
THE HEALTH FOR ALL PUBLISHING CO.

38, LANGHAM STREET, W.I

CONTENTS

ILLUSTRATIONS

PREFACE

THE human machine may be divided into four parts.

The part which feeds the machine and provides it with raw material is composed of the blood and the other liquids, the lymphatic ganglia, etc.

The second part, the nervous system, is the factory, which works by means of electro-magnetic currents. It takes in from the atmosphere what has been called the Prana or universal energy, accumulates this and transforms it into high frequency and low frequency according to the needs of the different organs.

The third part, the mental faculties, is an office, receiving all communications from outside and transmitting them to the brain, which sends back various kinds of orders. The accumulation of information thus acquired provides the fund of knowledge known as memory. The brain is the foreman in charge of the factory. His job is to maintain a state of equilibrium and normal distribution of labour, to keep all the different parts in order, to give orders to the workmen (for instance the arms), and finally to supervise external and internal cleansing.

The fourth part, the spiritual faculty, is the supreme directive power enabling the body to be conscious of its ultra-sensitive powers (manifested in such organs as the pineal gland), and to be aware of the accumulation of the ultra-sensitive vibrations of the universe, which feed the spirit, the heart, the and the body. When the human machine has developed its ultra-sensitive faculty to such a degree that it can feel the working of all the currents which pass through it, and can extend this realisation to a consciousness of the connection between these bodily vibrations and the ultra-sensitive vibrations of the whole universe — then true spirituality has been attained.

The wheels which set the machine in motion are the legs (which are workmen in the factory, like the arms and the hands). The headlights of the machine are the eyes, which guide its course and at the same time make visual observations. The examiner of air and food is the nose, which, before allowing the air to pass through it, filters it through the hairs which line it. The nose is also a kind of radiator which warms the air before it penetrates to the lungs, providing them with oxygen for the purification of the blood.

At the tip of the tongue is the sense of taste. Before allowing food to pass into the esophagus it analyses the taste. If normal, it sanctions; if bad, it rejects. But unfortunately humanity in general spoils this tip of the tongue by feeding it with too many irritating substances, with the result that it loses its power of selection and rejection, of discrimination between the nourishing and the poisonous. Similarly with the function of breathing; men rarely breathe through the nose. They are unaware that in breathing through the mouth they are ruining their throat and lungs, causing various kinds of afflictions, and even, sometimes, a most serious congestion which causes the stoppage of the machine, which is called death.

Next come the ears, which are a sort of telephone receiving station which registers every degree of sonority and passes on the information to the brain.

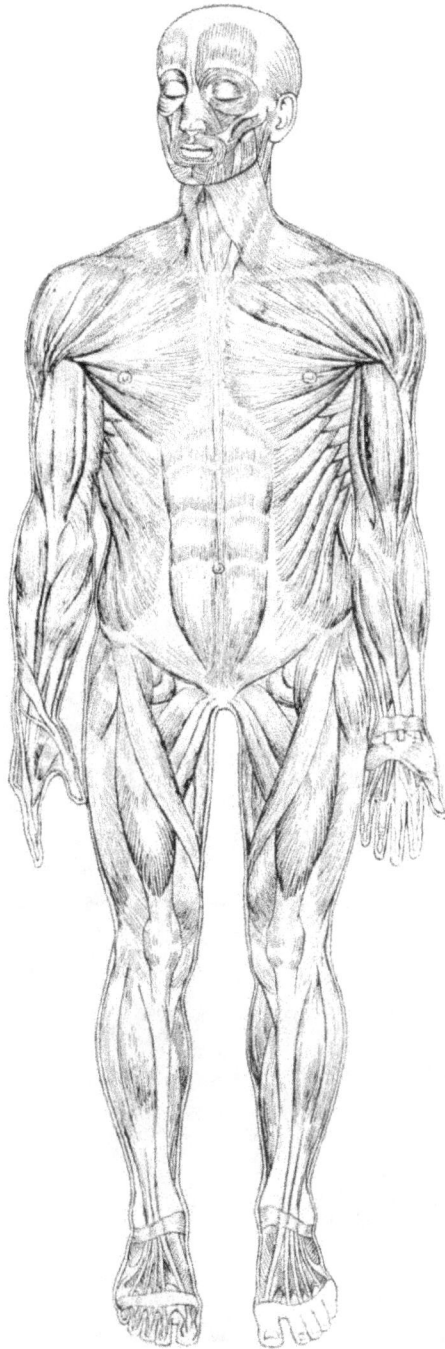

Fig. 1a
Muscular system of the body in its natural state (Front)

The sense of touch, which is not confined to any particular organ, records degrees of heat and cold, hardness and softness, etc.

Finally the brain, which is both creator and administrator, directs every movement by means of nervous and sensitive currents. It provides the whole machine with information, like an unseen and infallible Scotland Yard.

Together with the brain proper, we must include the ultra-sensitive faculties known variously as the soul, the spirit, the intellect and the consciousness. These faculties are as the king, the ministers and the judges of the human realm.

The whole system of creation comprises minerals, vegetables, animals and man. All are governed by a universal law, to which all the different functions must submit. The natural movement must prevail. If one or all the parts of the body create disorder, the mind cannot hold sway; just as it is impossible to command an army of disorderly soldiers, whilst it is possible for a single general to command thousands of well-conducted troops. If the machine is in good condition, everything works normally, and life goes on like a pleasant, happy journey. But with a disordered machine, there is not a second's pleasure or joy in life.

To take an illustration: if you buy a motor car, the salesman gives you a little booklet in which you find all sorts of explanations concerning the upkeep of the machine, how to feed it, when to clean it, when to overhaul it from chassis to engine, with a final admonition to examine the most important parts before starting up the car. You have a chauffeur or you drive yourself but in either case you must have a driving licence which you procure after passing a test.

But for the human machine, alas, there is no driving test, nobody bothers about it, there are no rules to direct and control its movements and to preserve its equilibrium. And if this lack of knowledge results in a disordered machine, there are neither garages, mechanics nor electricians capable of repairing the machine and putting it in normal working order.

Our aim is to create human garages throughout the world, and to give instruction to mechanics as to precise methods to be used in these human garages for the repairing of all kinds of disorders, whether they be physical, nervous or even mental.

CHAPTER 1
A SHORT HISTORY OF MEDICAL SCIENCE

THE earliest diagnoses were made by looking at the colour of the tongue, the eyes and the urine, and by feeling the pulsations of the blood at the wrist. In the same way modern diagnosis analyses the blood, the urine, the fecal matter, expectorations. The arterial tensions and the movements of the heart are examined, and methods such as cardiography, radiography and radioscopy are employed.

After diagnosis, follows treatment. We have studied almost all the generally accepted methods of cure for the various disorders of the human system.

Tracing back their history some seven thousand years, we discover the name of Dhanwantri, who has been called the Father of Medicine. The first inscriptions we find are the records of the method known as the Ayur Vedic.

The Ayur Vedic theory confines itself to treatment of the blood. All the remedies which it prescribes, whether animal, vegetable or mineral, are based on the precept that health is maintained by a just equilibrium of three forces, known as *vayu, pitte* and *kaf* (We may render these Sanskrit terms as roughly corresponding to air, fire and lymphatic substance.) If the patient reveals an excess of *kaf* the remedy is an increase of *pitte.* If the pitte is increased to an exaggerated extent, the remedy is an increase in strength of *kaf* and *vayu.* The three forces were thought to be confined solely to the liquid part of the body.

We cannot explain the Ayur Vedic method in detail — that would occupy several volumes — we are confining ourselves here simply to an explanation of its principles and scope in restoring health to the human body. The treatment began with a cleansing of the digestive tract by means of certain plants. Then mild purgatives were administered and light food in the form of various kinds of broth for the purification of the blood. Finally came the administration of ashes obtained by the oxidation of all kinds of minerals, from mica to copper, and also of certain plants. These ashes caused an artificial increase of appetite, induced digestion and aided assimilation.

There was also an athletic method of treatment known as the *Malla Vidia*. It was based on the game of "Catch As Catch Can." The patient, after a vigorous participation in this game, was massaged with oil to remove his general fatigue, and displaced bones in the spine were reset in position by the method of pounding with the feet. Accidents such as strained muscles, sprained or broken joints, were treated by an appropriate massage.

This method has been adopted by the Americans, who have ascribed to it certain scientific explanations and popularised it under the names of osteopathy and chiropractic.

The Ayur Vedic theory was taken over by Greece, with certain modifications in its application, resulting in the allopathic[1] form of treatment known as the Yoonanik, or Greek method. This method dispensed

---

1 Allopathy: [Greek, allos=other; pathos=disease]; Method of cure (followed by doctors today) by inducing an action contrary to that of the disease.

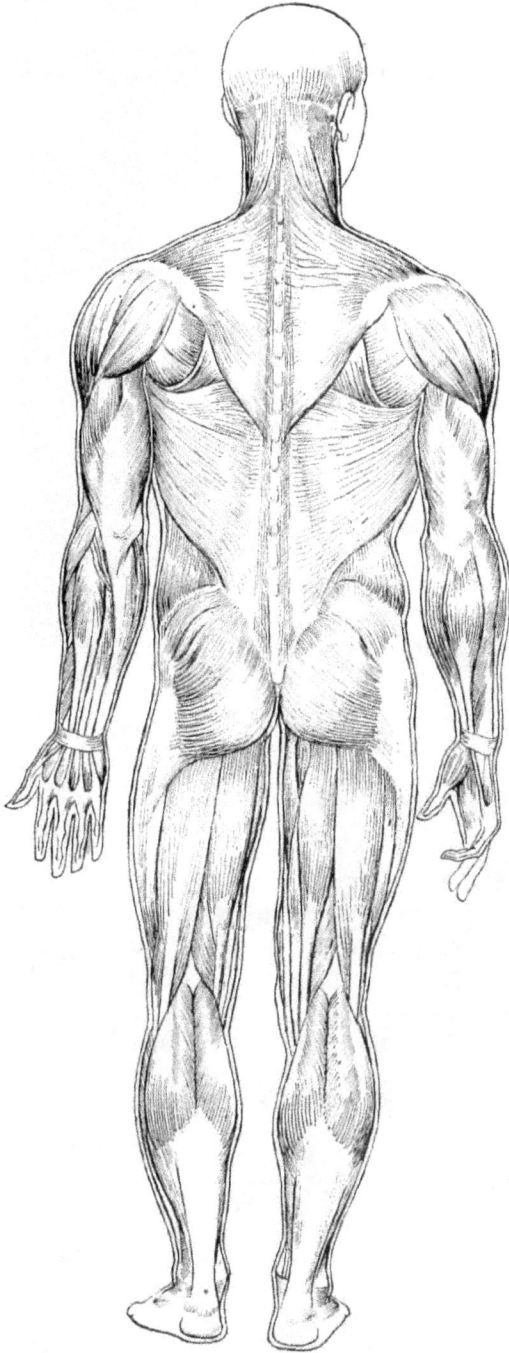

Fig. 1b
Muscular system of the body in its natural state (Back)

with the use of mineral ash, retaining that of vegetable matter, in the belief that all kinds of minerals are present in a transformed state in vegetables.[1] But the general principle remained the same: first, the cleansing of the digestive tract, then the purification of the blood and the prescription of appropriate food for the improvement of the blood stream. This method is chiefly concerned with the digestive system. Both methods are employed in the East to this day.

The Greek system of medicine extended to the rest of Europe, the principles, even the names of the maladies, remaining intact; but with the introduction of the use of certain medicaments. Various kinds of sera have been created for the benefit of the epicure who is averse to doses through the mouth.

Later, Pasteur contributed an allegedly "new" theory of microbes: that they enter the body from outside, and take up their residence within the body, which cannot be cured except by the destruction of these microbes.

The Ayur Vedic doctors knew of the existence of microbes, but did not seek to destroy them with medicaments. Their way was to increase the reproduction of blood by the method explained above, because a healthy and constantly renewed blood stream ensures a natural circulation free from microbes. In the same way a house which is not kept clean accumulates dirt, but as soon as it is swept and washed the dirt is forcibly eliminated.

The origin of microbes is fermentation. Wherever circulation becomes localised, the leucocytes and

1 Minerals (e. g., gold) have been reintroduced in modern allopathic treatment, particularly in the form of salts.

phagocytes are hemmed in, stagnate, and become deformed. If they are examined through the microscope and analysed, these leucocytes and phagocytes are seen to have assumed the form of what are known as microbes. Occasionally, during epidemics, microbes enter the body from the outside, but they accumulate only in parts where the blood has become localised.

In 1924, after having experimented on our theory, Professor Tissot, in the National Laboratory of Paris, confirmed it as exact. He took all kinds of vegetables, sterilised them and enclosed them in sealed jars which no microbe could penetrate from the outside. Some time after, when these vegetables had fermented, it was discovered that the carrots, the potatoes, the cauliflower, etc., contained microbes of cholera and other diseases.

The Professor communicated his findings to the Paris Academy of Medicine.

We ourselves have proceeded further to research into the cause of fermentation. We have discovered that the circulation of the nervous currents, which distributes heat proportionally throughout the whole organism, slows down occasionally because of the obstruction caused by certain adhesions; the muscular fibres harden together and the nervous currents can no longer pass through them, the supply of heat is reduced, the arteries harden, the blood thickens and its distribution slows down or stops completely.

Where the flow of blood and lymphatic liquid fails to be renewed, fermentation begins. Gradually the fermented matter begins to reveal microbes. Thus we have demonstrated both theoretically and. practically that the microbe theory is merely an indication of the real cause of the malady, *i.e.*, some disorder in the circulation of the nervous current.

It has been discovered that microbes can be killed by means of certain sera. This may be true, but local disorder can be traced to disorder in the circuit of nervous currents. No serum can adjust the nervous system, that is why we have sought to treat those currents directly.

We must not conclude without mentioning another method, which is practised throughout the world under the name of Homeopathy. This is based on the theory of the vibrations of the human body and of the vegetable and mineral world. To maintain the equilibrium of these vibrations, buccal administration in minute doses of remedies which act upon the circulation of the blood is employed.

There is also electro-therapy, the treatment by means of coloured light rays and high frequency (diathermy). Electrotherapy is particularly useful in healing wounds and in eliminating excessive fat. Diathermy gives temporary aid to the circulation by means of artificial heat.

Surgery has made great progress, particularly in the transfusion of blood, which has saved many lives, and in the removal of completely shattered limbs.

Finally, Nature Cure, which follows the general principles of the old Ayur Vedic and Yoonanik schools — removal of intoxication of the blood stream by means of special diet, fresh air and exercise, combined with rest for the nervous and digestive systems. It differs from the old form of treatment in its use of modern devices such as the colon douche, and of modern sanatorium equipment.

There are methods of suggestion and auto-suggestion based on the use of mental force through individual and collective prayer. We agree that results can be achieved through faith, but, it is also our opinion that God gave us for our use not only a mind, hut hands and a mouth, too, by the aid of which we can restore our bodies when anything goes wrong. If by eating or drinking certain things we can restore the nervous equilibrium of the body, or remove any toxic matter from it, we are not forbidden to do so by God. On the contrary, by acting in this way we are assisting the working of the universal law of creation.

In our twenty-two years of practice we have demonstrated effective and positive methods designed to restore nervous equilibrium which promotes the healthy circulation of the blood, so that new tissues begin to be built, up again. Not only is the affected part regenerated, but the whole body is renewed. This may indeed be called a restoration of health.

Any obstruction in the flow of nervous current is a hindrance to the carrying out of the universal law of creation. Our method of treatment by the removal of all obstacles to the flow of nervous current (*Pranotherapy*) allows creation to proceed unimpeded.

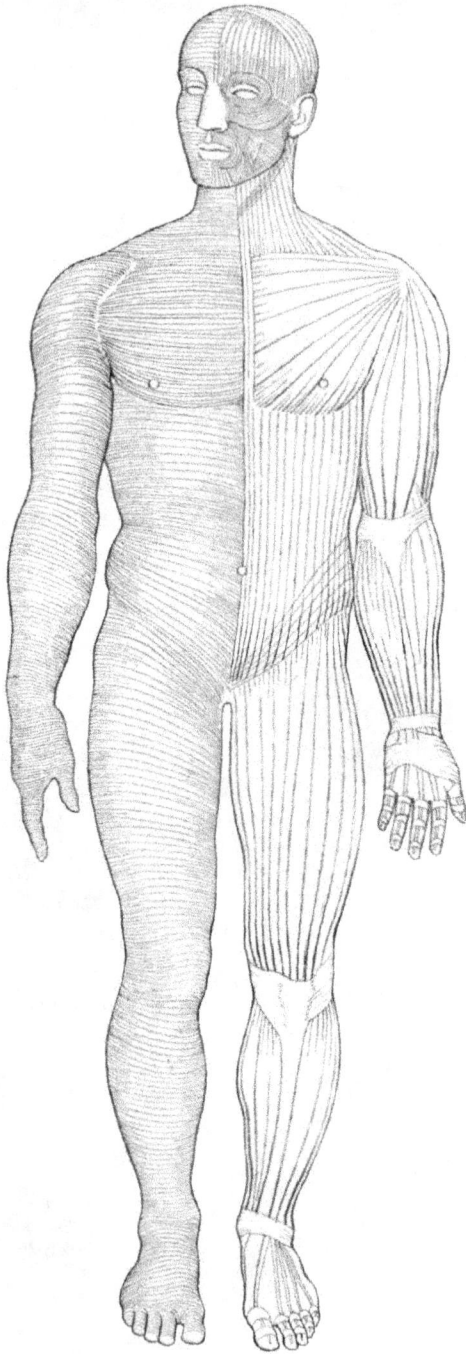

Fig. 2a

The passage of the nervous current throughout the body
from head to foot The curved lines on the left, indicate
the spiral stream of current which passes through the
nerve-fibres underlying the superficial muscles, providing
the surface of the body with warmth and sensitivity.
The vertical lines on the right indicate the downward
passage of the current through the nerve-fibres underlying the deep-seated muscles providing the power of
contraction and relaxation. (Front)

Chapter 11
THE NERVOUS SYSTEM

IN the course of long years of research and practice we have sought to discover the law of creation.

This is our conclusion:

Variation of vibration is the cause of creation

Vibration is the manifestation and movement of life - it is life itself. The source of all vibration is the universal force known as the Prana, of which the most, tangible manifestations are the ultra-sensitive currents of the atmosphere, whose function we shall endeavour to explain in the course of these chapters.

For a, long time scientists have known, and made use of, the electric currents of the atmosphere, under the general title of electricity, and, more recently, as Hertzian waves and electromagnetic vibrations. A few years ago a Belgian scientist discovered ultra-penetrating vibrations ten miles up in the atmosphere. Many kinds of atmospheric currents are in common use, providing light, motive power, wireless telegraphy, telephony, telephotography, television, etc.

All these different manifestations of vibratory energy are dependent upon varying degrees of high frequency and low frequency. Yet, although these currents are used in such diverse ways, it is maintained that their origin is unknown.

To understand all the currents of the atmosphere, their source and their function, one must employ the scientific method of the Yoga, the observation and study of the ultra-sensitive vibrations of the Prana. It was by this method that we arrived at the conclusion formulated above: variation of vibration is the cause of creation.

All the forms manifested in the universe, whether visible or invisible, are based on innumerable variations of vibrations, We have discovered by means of our apparatus for measuring vibrations (the Pranograph)[1] that a pigeon registers 720 vibrations per second. All birds have a higher rate of vibration than other animals. In the animal kingdom we find the lowest number of vibrations in the tortoise (18 per second) and the snail (18 per second). The vegetable kingdom has the lowest rate of all.

But we are concerned here solely with the human mechanism. The average number of vibrations for man is 860 per second, the proportion being much higher in the head than in the feet. Thus varying degrees of high frequency and low frequency can be recorded throughout the body from the top of the head to the tips of the fingers and toes. Just as a river descends from the mountains, feeding the land. through which it passes, and flows out to the ocean, so all kinds of currents enter our bodies at the head, nourish all our organs as they pass through them, and flow out through our hands and feet. In this way life is continually renewed.

These currents provide the body with varying degrees of heat in order to regulate the density of its fluid content. When the heat is increased, the blood and the other liquids become thinner, and vice versa. We find

1 See concluding sections of this chapter,.

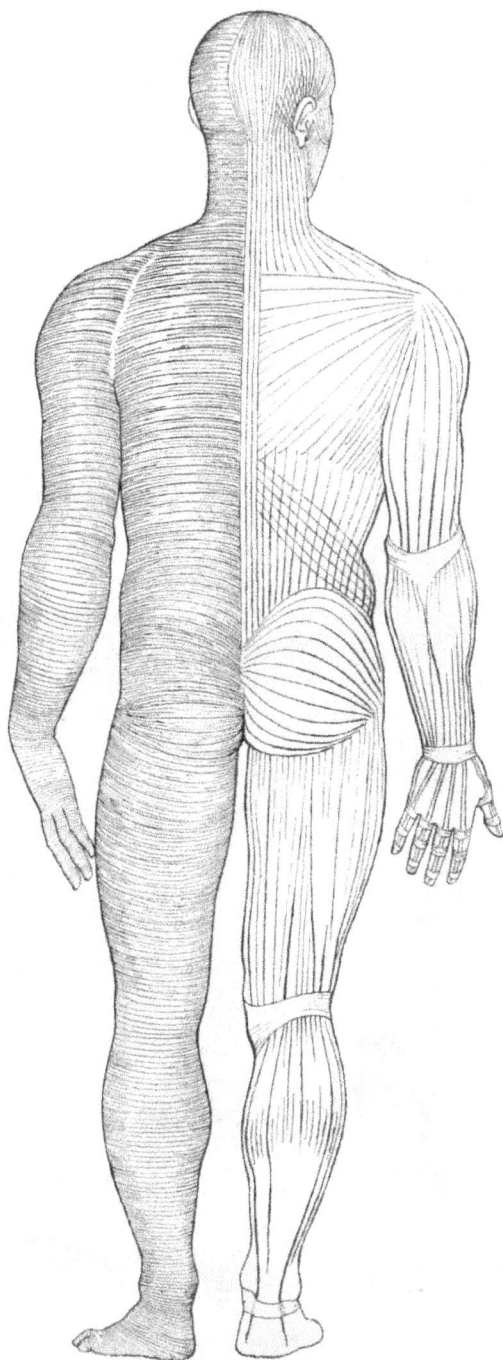

Fig. 2b

As Fig 2a   (Back)

the maximum temperature just below the medulla oblongata, in the first cervical vertebra (the Atlas), and the minimum temperature at the tips of the fingers and toes.

To these variations of temperature correspond variations of texture of the nerve fibres through which the currents pass; in the head and the upper part of the body we find very thin fibres, and in the arms and lower parts the fibres are thicker and longer, We can best explain this by a comparison with the law of sound vibrations: the long, thick chords produce low notes, and the short, thin chords produce high notes — the difference in quality corresponding to difference in texture, It is at the joints particularly that we note changes of thickness in the nerve fibres, and to this we may correlate the fact that the currents are transformed at the joints and distributed to the different parts of the body,

The Distribution of the Nervous Current

How does the human body intercept these currents, whose vibrations emanate from the primordial energy of the universe (the Prana), and which are the source of its creation and renewal?

We have discovered that our bodies pick up two kinds of currents at two points: the ultra-sensitive currents at the pineal gland, and the sensitive currents at the nerve fibres below the cranium.

The ultra-sensitive currents create the invisible faculties — the soul, the spirit, the heart, the consciousness and the mind. The latter includes all the various mental forces such as the reasoning power, the memory, the analytical faculty and the directive forces which control the information agencies communicating to the brain all that happens to the body. The sensitive currents create the bodily tissues and provide the body with fuel and motive power in the form of heat. and muscular contraction.

The ultra-sensitive vibrations, starting from the pineal gland in the middle of the encephalus, pursue a circular route, passing through back and front, (spinal cord and sternum) to the middle of the body.

This produces a kind of circuit with two poles, the pineal gland and the coccygeal plexus.[1] Between these two poles the currents flow downwards to stimulate the different organs, and upwards to inform the brain of' heat or cold, pain or over-sensitivity. The stoppage of circulation in any part, irritation or other pathological phenomena such as indigestion, stiffness of joints and all the ailments of a disordered nervous system — every form of abnormal condition is communicated to the brain by the returning flow of sensitive currents.

The sensitive vibrations, after being received in the nerve fibres below the cranium, are condensed in the cerebellum, which contains a substance which acts like an accumulator. The cerebellum is a kind of induction coil which produces heat and distributes it by way of the medulla oblongata and the spinal cord. As we have already indicated. one stream of this current flows from the cerebellum along the nerve fibres throughout the body, transforming itself at the joints and passing out of the body at the tips of the fingers and toes. Another

1.The Sanskrit *brhamand* (universal egg) is applied to the pineal gland, and the Sanskrit *swastika* to the coccygeal plexus.

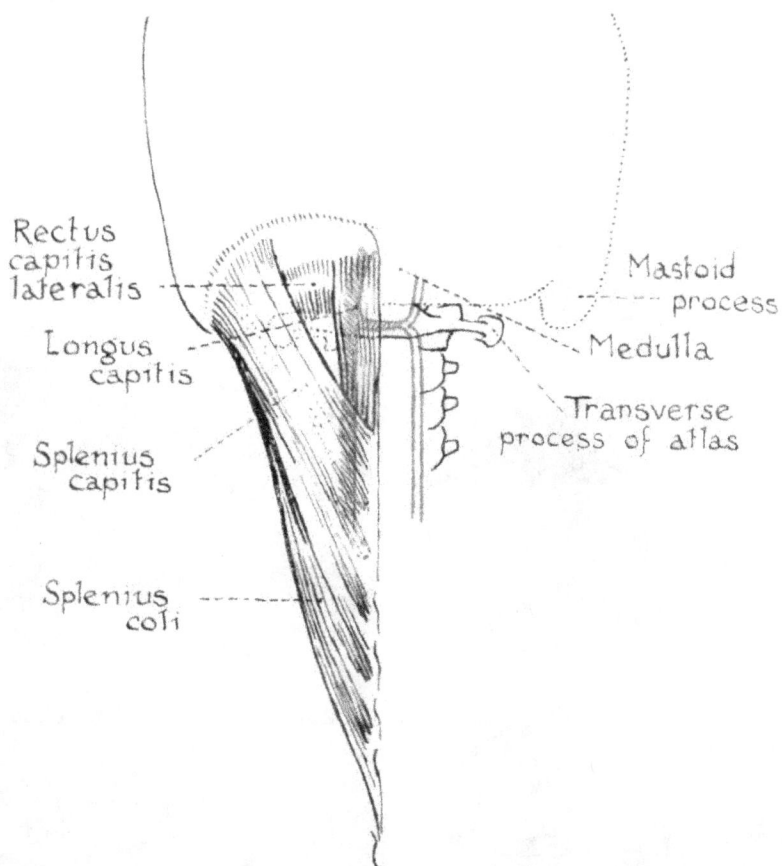

Rectus
capitis
lateralis

Longus
capitis

Splenius
capitis

Splenius
coli

Mastoid
process

Medulla

Transverse
process of atlas

Fig. 3.

Diagram showing the position of the Atlas at the base
of the skull. On the left are shown the overlying
muscular fivers: if these become permanently
contracted the outlet of the nervous current is blocked. (See
Chapter II)

stream begins its course on either side of the Atlas (the first cervical vertebra) and flows round the body in a continuous spiral motion. If adhesions of muscular fibres occur in the region of the Atlas, this current cannot pass easily, and the body suffers from the deficiency. In cases of very obstructive adhesions it is cut off just as in the case of a "blown " electric fuse, and the body dies.

On either side of the spinal column, from the Atlas to the coccyx, we find sympathetic nerve ganglia, which are protected by muscular fibres. These ganglia act as electric batteries which are charged with the descending current and which distribute this current to right and left to the various organs. (*See illustration*)

The nerve-cells all over the body act both as accumulators and non- conductors of the nervous current passing through the nerve fibres. The cervical plexus and the solar plexus possess a great many nerve cells, because they both need plentiful supplies of heat, the former for the creation of the delicate tissues of the sense-organs, and the latter to assist the functioning of the digestive organs. The masses of nerve cells on the breasts play an important part in the provision of heat to the organs of the thorax.

Subsequent chapters will describe more fully the function of the nervous currents and their vital importance in the treatment of disease. It will suffice to conclude this description with a general indication of their activity. For instance, special mention way well be made of the sensitive current which is to be found in the first of the four layers of the skin. If the latter is in normal condition, the nervous current passes freely through the nerve fibres, but if the skin becomes attached to the underlying muscle, the current cannot pass, the part loses its sensibility and is said to be paralysed.

Again, the motor and thermic currents control the contraction and relaxation of the muscles and the creation of all kinds of tissues, which in the neck and head are very fine, but at the tips of the fingers and toes are very thick and condensed, especially in the nails. The tissues of the bones are even more closely knit, so that they are completely hard.

In the next chapter we shall deal more fully with the formation of the bodily tissues; we have confined ourselves here to a mere statement of the existence of thermic and motor currents and of their varying degrees of sensitivity.

The Pranograph

During the last twelve years we have constructed several kinds of apparatus. Finally, we have succeeded in producing an apparatus to which we have given the name of Pranograph. The Pranograph picks up the low frequency vibratory currents engendered in the human body by the primordial vibration (Prana), and amplifies them twelve million times. It photographs on highly sensitive films the vibrations of all the different parts of the body, at the same time enabling the operator to hear the varying sonority of the vibrations and to count the number of vibrations per second.

The apparatus gives one a clear indication of the state in which the various organs are functioning.

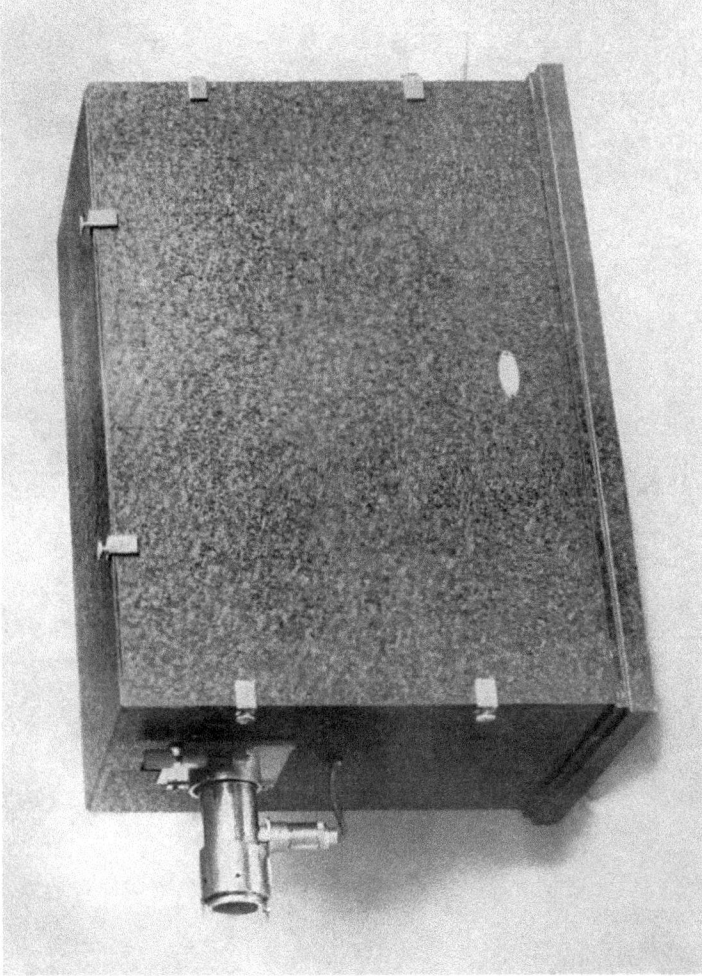

Fig. 4a The Pranograph

In a normally constituted individual the vibrations should be very regular and of average amplitude. If they become irregular and of high amplitude, it means that there is an accumulation of current in the organ in question, which is functioning badly in consequence. If, on the other hand, the vibrations, although regular, are of low amplitude, it means that the current is insufficient; it has accumulated elsewhere and must be traced back to its source.

The Pranograph is thus an infallible instrument of diagnosis, revealing not only the particular organ which is affected, but also the actual cause of the affection and the progress of its cure in the course of treatment.

It is a very necessary means of control and checking-up of conditions before and after pranotherapeutic treatment, for people to-day are skeptical of results until they have seen a scientific demonstration of proof.

The Pranometer is an apparatus which tests the findings of the Pranograph, lt deals with the heat of the bodily fibres. By means of a special kind of thermometer it records the temperature of the different, parts of the body. Thus, if the Pranograph gives evidence of any disorder in the vibrations of any particular part, the Pranometer verifies this disorder by demonstrating whether the temperature of this particular part is normal or not. If the temperature is abnormal. the number of vibrations must be abnormal, and vice versa.

Chapter III
HOW TISSUES ARE FORMED

W E find that the body is composed of tissues which vary in texture from head to foot in accordance with the needs of the various organs and muscles. There are delicate and supple tissues like those of the ear, and progressively coarser and more resistant tissues until we reach the bones, which are the carcass or basic structure of the dwelling.

Where it is necessary to produce fine, supple tissues, the heat of the nervous vibrations is increased, for at higher temperatures the blood has a finer fluid content. In places where the functions of the body require fairly thick, or completely hard tissues, the heat is decreased proportionately,

We have already indicated that the body in its normal state has a minimum heat firstly at the tips of the toes and secondly at the tips of the fingers. After each joint the temperature is increased by one degree centigrade, until the maximum of about 33"C. is reached in the medulla oblongata. (At the fingertips it is only about 25°C.) This proves that the heat is produced by the nervous system, and not by the blood, as the medical world maintains. If the latter were the case, either we should find the maximum heat at the heart, whereas the temperature of the heart is 35"C., or else, as the blood is present in all parts of the body, these variations of heat would not exist at all.

The purpose of this variation of heat is to keep the blood in a more or less liquid state, If the blood stream

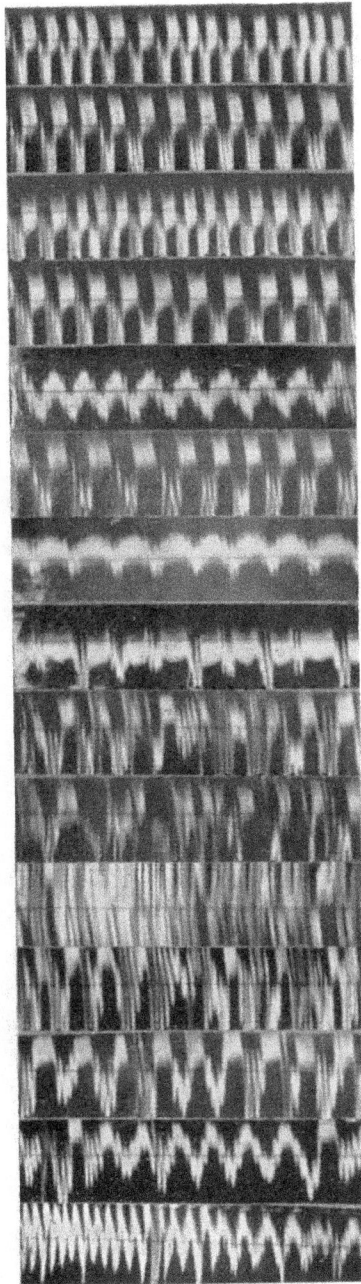

Fig. 4b.   Vibrations of an unhealthy body photographed by the Pranograph. Note the serious disorders in the lower limbs.
(varicose veins)

and the nervous current are circulating normally, they go on manufacturing tissues as we manufacture cloth in a silk, cotton or jute textile mill. Textures as fine as muslin or as coarse as matting are woven in these mills. The fine materials are made with fine threads or fibres, and the coarse materials with coarse ones, The same thing happens in the human body, The delicate layers of the skin are made up of fine fibres; but the sheaths covering the nervous fibres are in parts so fine that they have to be magnified at least a thousand times to enable them to be seen. What a marvelous piece of natural manufacture!

More tissues are formed in parts which are more quickly worn away. Organs like the ear-drum, which undergo very little friction, are renewed much more slowly, as the tissues last much longer here.

It is a matter of common experience that where any part of the body is scratched or torn or cut, the process of reproduction begins at once and a scar is quickly formed. For example, a man cuts himself while shaving. Three minutes later he thinks the cut has healed up, but. this is not the case. The broken tissues have merely formed a protective crust which remains until the new tissues are ready to take their place on the surface of the skin. Then the old tissues are discarded, leaving such a wonderful piece of mending that even with a microscope no trace of a wound is to be seen.

But if the blood stream or the nervous currents are not flowering normally, the cicatrice is badly made and traces of the wound remain for the rest of the patient's life. Similarly with broken bones, which with some people heal in a week, and with others never heal at all. When sugar is deposited in the blood-stream, the blood becomes incapable of manufacturing tissues, so that it is very difficult to heal cuts and broken bones of sufferers from advanced diabetes. We have known of diabetics who have died as the result of simple wounds.

When the formation of tissues slows down, it is generally a sign of old age. Fewer vibrations are picked up, and the ligaments of all the vertebrae harden, especially the two muscles on either side of the vertebra which protect the hyper-sympathetic nerve ganglia. The distribution of currents slows down in all the organs, the tissues fail to be renewed and gradually the functioning power of the various organs is weakened, causing arteriosclerosis (hardening of the arteries). Lack of moisture is everywhere manifest, as in a garden which loses its supply of rain-water, so that the plants in it gradually fade and die.

If in a certain part of the body the tissues are insufficiently reproduced, the organ in question weakens and is finally paralysed. Sometimes the circulation in a certain organ stops, and the organ ferments. The fermentation produces microbes, which generate disease. If this disease is not checked in time, the fermentation becomes general and leads to the stoppage of the machine, in other words, to death.

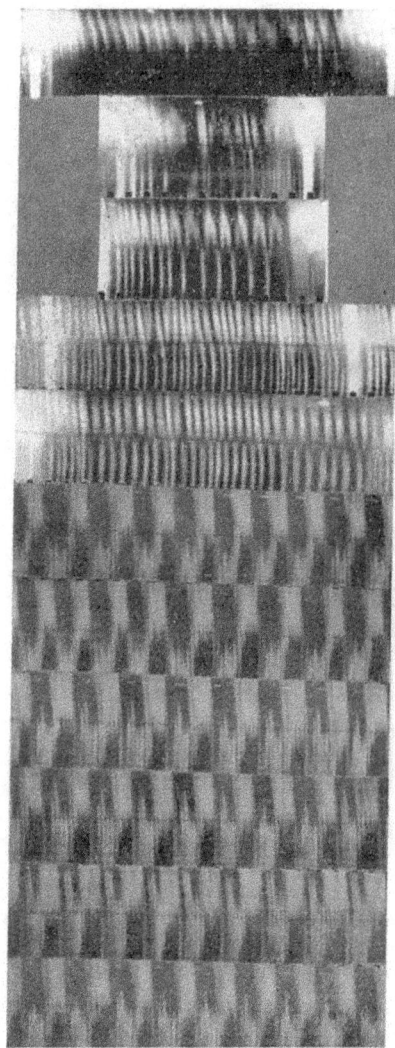

Fig. 4c   As Fig. 4b Note the
disorder in the upper part of
the body. (Headaches)

Chapter IV
THE CIRCULATORY SYSTEM

ALL factories need raw materials, and the raw material of the body is the blood. The average body contains about five litres of blood; if the body is small it contains rather less blood, if large the amount is proportionally increased. As the factory goes on producing various kinds of tissues, the blood is used up, and it must be replaced. The distillery of the blood is the digestive tract.

How do we manufacture fresh blood ?

As we have indicated above, we renew our blood supply in the process of eating. We partake of all kinds of food, taking it first into the mouth, where if it is solid, it is masticated by the teeth and mingled with saliva, which is secreted by the salivary glands. As long as the food remains in the mouth during mastication the saliva continues to be mixed with it. The regular and proportional swallowing of saliva is a great help to the digestion.

After being masticated, the food passes down the esophagus to the stomach, and thence via the pylorus to the duodenum, where it receives the secretions of the liver and the pancreas, and becomes bitter in taste. In the jejunum (the second part of the small intestine) there are thousands of glands, whose secretions change the taste again to an insipid flavour. In the third part of the small intestine (the ileum) the glandular secretions render the taste of the food sweet and slightly salt.

When its digestion is completed, the food is filtered by means of a kind of valve which extracts from it a fine liquid known as chyle, which is conveyed along the thoracic duct directly to the superior vena cava beside the clavicle.

The remainder is passed into the large intestine, where it is rendered less dry by a secretion from a gland known as the appendix, which assists in the evacuation of faecal matter. (We have noted that persons without appendices have a tendency to constipation.) After being thus softened by the appendix, this solid residue of digested food is pushed forward by the air which enters the mouth during every process of swallowing, and is finally evacuated through the rectum.

How we use the blood

Various organs play an important part in the circulatory system of the body.

The *spleen* is a major factor in the formation of the red corpuscles. When the blood circulates through the *lungs,* these red corpuscles take up oxygen from the lungs, which are thus responsible for the purification and changing of colour of the blood.

The *bronchial tubes* act as electrical resisters, providing the lungs and the heart with necessary heat from the nervous vibrations. The current is accumulated in the bronchial tubes, just as an electrical current is accumulated in the spiral tubes inside an electric radiator, iron, etc.

The *heart* plays a double part, receiving the venous blood, transforming it into arterial blood and sending it

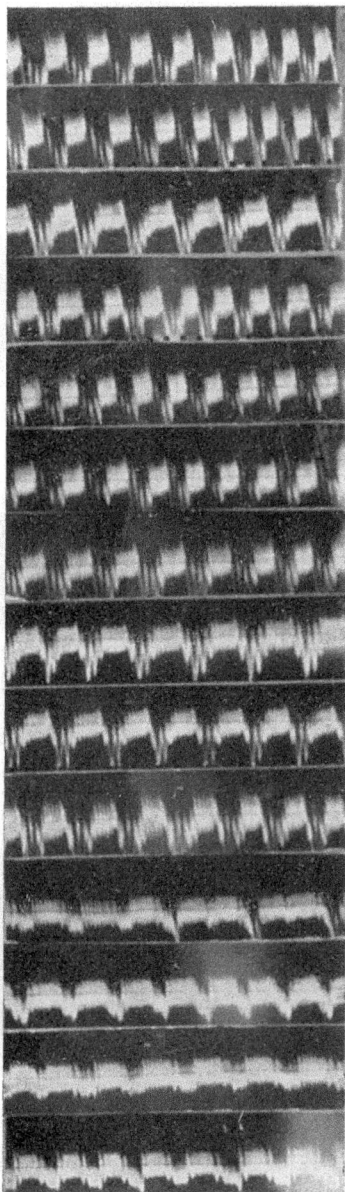

Fig. 4d.   Vibrations of a healthy
body.   Note the regularity of
     the vibratory curves.

back to the lungs and to all the different parts of the body in regular and automatic distribution through the large artery known as the aorta.

The *spinal cord* contains liquids which protect the nervous and sensitive fibres. The marrow contained in the bones prevents them from getting too dry.

The lymphatic fluid

The lymphatic ganglia are formed and preserved in that part of the body which lies beneath the navel. The lymphatic fluid also circulates throughout the body. Its chief function is connected with the joints. It feeds the synovial fluid which lubricates the joints, together with the bony tissues, the ligaments and the cartilages. The lymphatic ganglia also assist the functioning of the glands, providing them with raw material to be transformed into glandular secretions. The lymphatic fluid feeds the glands, and under the influence of the heat of the nervous currents, this fluid is transformed into the different glandular secretions; for instance, into saliva for the salivary glands, etc. It has also the function of bathing the veins, arteries, fibres, etc., so that they remain separated and do not adhere in any way.

The acid and other liquid refuse from these different processes is filtered by the kidneys and evacuated by the bladder, besides being eliminated by perspiration through the pores of the skin.

How we should nourish the blood

If the body is being supplied with clean and wholesome food, in proper balance, and all the organs are functioning normally, the blood remains pure, and the organic and muscular tissues remain supple and constantly renewed.

But if the food is impure and unbalanced in its constituents, or if large quantities of meat are eaten, the tissues will lose their suppleness and become tough. More meat is eaten in cold countries, and it is in these countries that cancer is more prevalent. The diet should be moderate and balanced, with plenty of vegetables. Animal, vegetable and mineral substances to supply the needs of all the different parts of the organism should be taken in proportions adapted to the climate and the nature of one's work. But there must be no excess of any kind of nourishment, Exaggerated quantities, even of good food, are as poison. The organs and glands can perform only a limited amount of work: if they are given too much to do they can neither digest nor assimilate. This is the cause of intoxication.

Thus each person should adjust his diet to his own constitution and expenditure of energy (a ten-horse-power motor needs less petrol than a forty). Then his blood stream will be pure and his tissues supple.

Why do we need to eat'? As a rule people eat when they are hungry, and the feeling of hunger is caused by the contraction of the stomach when it is empty. If the stomach remains empty it often feels cramped until it is re-distended with food. Rut actually this "hunger" is merely a way of manifesting a more vital need of the body — the need to renew the supply of raw material for the manufacture of fresh blood and consequently of fresh tissues.

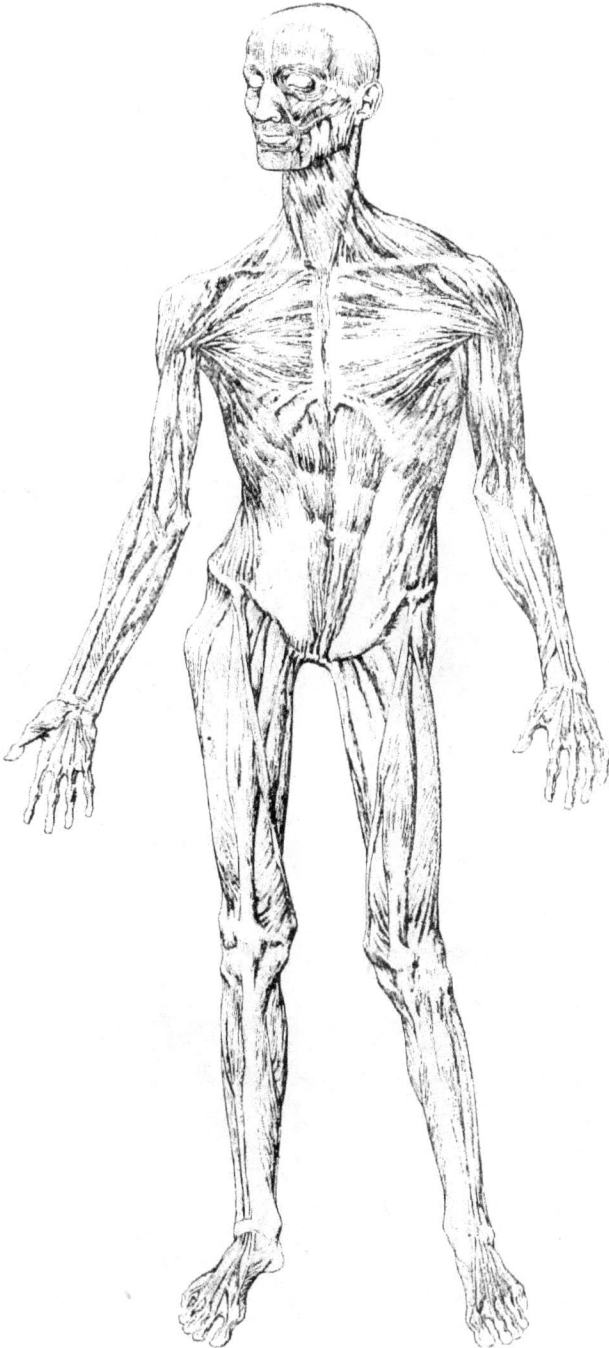

Fig. 5a.
Muscular Atrophy

When an inadequate supply of nervous current is taken
in at the head. The distribution of the current *via* the
Atlas, the spinal cord and the sternum slows down, and
the creation of fresh tissues is reduced. This leads to
partial or general muscular atrophy. Note the deform-
aion of the joints. (front)

If the quality of the raw material is good, the quality of the finished product, (in this case the bodily tissues) will be equally good. Hence the importance of eating the best and most suitable kinds of food.

The kind and the amount of food required depends on the climatic conditions. In hot countries the body receives nourishment directly from the rays of the sun, and in the same way the fruits and vegetables which grow there acquire concentrated nourishing properties from these rays, Therefore, in these countries man has no difficulty in feeding himself on the natural fruits of the earth. For instance, in the Sahara there is an abundance of dates (which are ten times more nourishing than meat), goat's milk and water melons (the rind of which is eaten by the camels!). In rather cooler countries we find, for instance, that the staple food is lentils of various kinds, which are rich in mineral salts — there are yellow lentils which contain gold, black lentils which contain iron, white lentils which contain silver, red lentils which contain copper, etc.— all of which provide the body with nourishment and vitality.

Heat causes loss of appetite, which means a reduction in the appropriate glandular secretion; hence the prevalence in these parts of all kinds of pimentos and hot condiments, which " tickle the palate " and stimulate secretion by the glands. Toxic matter is evacuated through the perspiration induced by these spices. A great deal of rice is eaten with this highly spiced food, so that its heating property is reduced. It is commendable that in these hot, countries vegetables are usually cooked in their own juice.

But in cold countries the fruits of the earth are less affected by the life-giving properties of the sun's rays. Vegetables are for the most part water, yet it is customary in these countries to boil these vegetables in more water, with the result that what vital forces they contain — the life blood of the vegetable — are drawn out into the water, and all that is eaten is the refuse.

Meat, poultry and fish are also important parts of the diet in cold countries. Fish has a lower number of vibrations than other animals, and is therefore easier to digest. Vegetables have a still lower number of vibrations. Meat having a comparatively high vibration value should not form more that a small part of the diet.

In cold countries, the inside of the body is warm relatively to external conditions (the reverse is the case in hot countries), therefore the digestion does not need to be stimulated by spices, which would induce excessive glandular secretion. Neither should the appetite be stimulated artificially by aperitifs and cocktails, nor the digestion " assisted " by after-dinner liqueurs, which condemn the natural functions of the stomach to death. If the appetite and the digestive process need some stimulus, this must be provided by exercises and particularly by correct breathing, as a fire is stimulated by bellows.

We repeat that the body should be nourished according to climate and digestive powers. Nature must never be forced. Food must be absorbed to suit the occupation and temperament of the individual. The spiritual type of person, who docs not consume much physical energy, should eat very light, vital food, such as

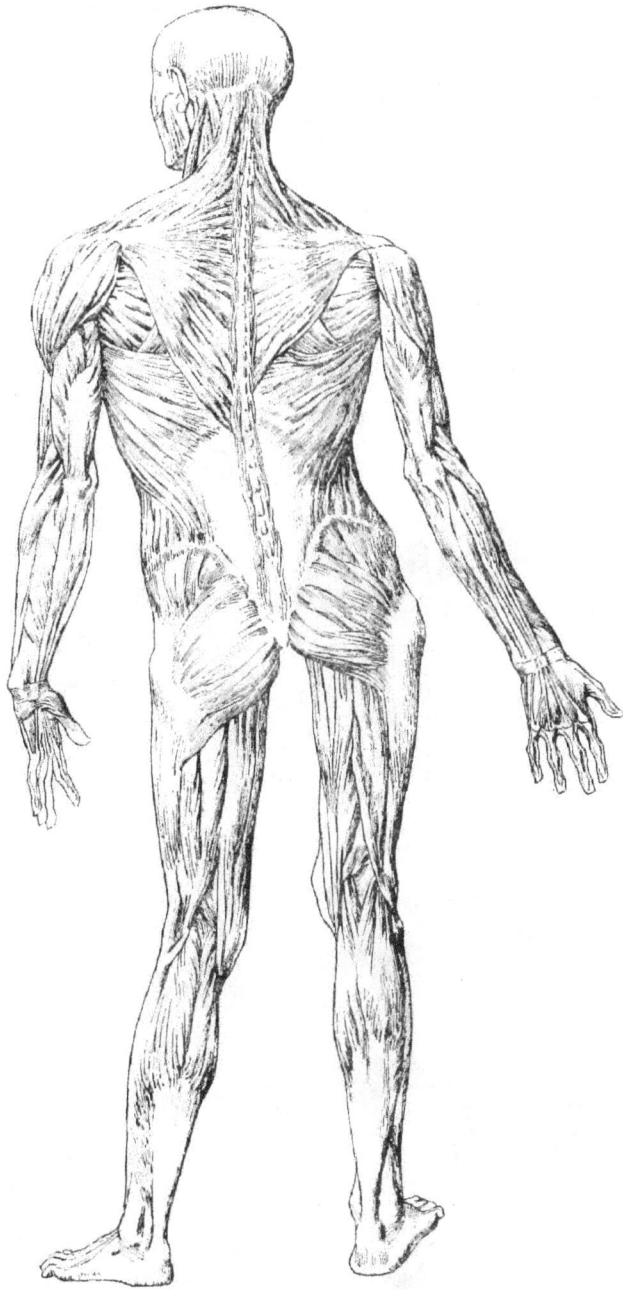

Fig. 5b.

Muscular atrophy as Fig. 5a   (back)

ground almonds with honey or sugar, to fortify the brain and central nervous system. vegetables, ripe (but not over ripe) fruit, milk, butter and cream. Intellectuals need a similar diet, with the addition of cereals and more concentrated food such as lentils, and poultry, meat and fish in small quantities (provided the climate is cool enough). The greater the person's activity, the greater the number of vibrations he requires to assimilate in the form of food. Manual workers need more cereals, lentils and meat, and the physical exercise which they take enables them to digest these easily.

Speaking of digestion, we are reminded of the importance of the use of the teeth and saliva. If food is well masticated, half the digestion is completed in the mouth; if pieces of food are swallowed whole, the poor stomach, which has no teeth, has to expel this undigested food as best it can, This causes constipation, which in turn may lead to appendicitis. If a piece of this undigested food becomes lodged in a curve of the intestine it may ferment and generate microbes of intestinal tuberculosis, enteritis, etc.

Food must never be eaten merely to satisfy the sense of taste, which should not dominate the process of nutrition, but serve it by examining the quality of the food before it is swallowed. The amount of food taken should be strictly limited to ensure that the stomach is never over-full, for it must have room to contract in order to mix the glandular secretions with the food contained in it. Over-eating is another cause of constipation. The waste part of the digested food should be naturally evacuated twice daily, at morning and night, and at least one evacuation per day is absolutely essential to a healthy body, But medicaments which promote forcible evacuation are harmful to the natural glandular functioning of the intestines. If food is eaten in the way we have described, constipation and fermentation will be impossible. An occasional flushing of the bowel with oil and water is quite useful as a lubricant, but if it is allowed to become a habit, the walls of the intestine dilate and the glands have difficulty in secreting.

Very little drink should be taken with food, unless this is very dry. But the blood stream must be kept clean, so that a glass of fresh water should be drunk every morning and two hours after every meal. As a rule at least two quarts of water are required daily for the thorough cleansing of the blood, kidneys and bladder. More liquid is needed in summer than in winter. It must be remembered that soup, tea, etc., also contain water; but pure water. is the best drink of all. In cold countries, cider and a little light wine are permissible, but habitual drinking of excessive quantities of alcohol causes the blood to deteriorate, creates very hard tissues, and consequently promotes various kinds of disease. This shows the folly of drinking, whether through vice or through "politeness," at the risk of deranging the whole human mechanism.

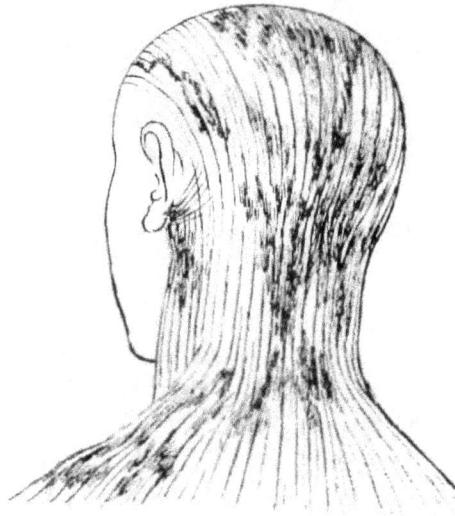

Fig. 6a.

Affections of the head and neck.

Adhesions in the upper part of the head, preventing the
assimilation of sufficient vibratory currents from the
atmosphere. Adhesions at the base of the skull and in
the neck prevent the free passage of nervous currents
from the Atlas. Adhesions below the ears causing head
noises and deafness. Adhesions at the shoulders causing
all kinds of afflictions of the arms and fingers

CHAPTER V
HOW WE FALL ILL

WE have already declared this human machine to be a marvel of marvels, indeed the source of all other marvels; and since men have existed in the world they have studied themselves in the measure of their capacity, their observation and their knowledge, under the title of demigods, sons of gods, prophets, saints, philosophers, founders of religions, and finally Viadias (Hindu doctors), Tubibs (Arab doctors), Hakims (Persian doctors) and European medical men.

All these different categories of men have made a study of the human body; but none till now has produced a clear and simple exposition of theory as to its creation and function. We find the most detailed study of this question in the works of the Yogis. The science of Yoga deals with the Prana, or nervous currents, which are said to be creative, ultra-penetrating and universal. All forms, all colours, all visible and invisible substances are created by the Prana.

But how and by what means does the Prana create *diversity* of form? How is the varied and proportionate nourishment and renewal of all forms and substances carried out? We have found no answer to this either in the Patanjali or in any of the other writings of the Yogis. Only after long years of research and practical experience in dealing with the human body, particularly our own, have we discovered the law of creation enunciated in a previous chapter: variation of vibration is the cause of creation. That is to say, the primordial, ultra-sensitive vibrations (the Prana) create every kind of substance according to their presence in greater or lesser number; for example, whilst the colour red is achieved by nine hundred vibrations to the second, the colour blue requires eight hundred. The *number* of vibrations changes, but the vibrations themselves do not change their original substance. To use the language of electricity, the vibrations assume different forms as a result of different degrees of high frequency and low frequency. Short and long waves, whether atmospheric or other, are formed of the same kind of vibrations in different degrees of acceleration. Rapid vibrations produce short waves, slow vibrations produce long waves, but the vibrations themselves do not change anything but their speed.

To continue our recapitulation; the human mechanism, created by these same vibrations, is fed according to climatic conditions by all kinds of mineral elements condensed in vegetable produce and transformed in animal matter. It is provided with motive power and heat to assist the regular distribution of the blood, and with a system of respiration (abdominal, thoracic and mental) by which it maintains the vital nervous current in a state of equilibrium. (With the mind and other superior forces governing the human machine we will deal more fully in studies which we have in preparation on physical, nervous and mental education.)

We must now return to the practical application of this new understanding of the creation and functioning

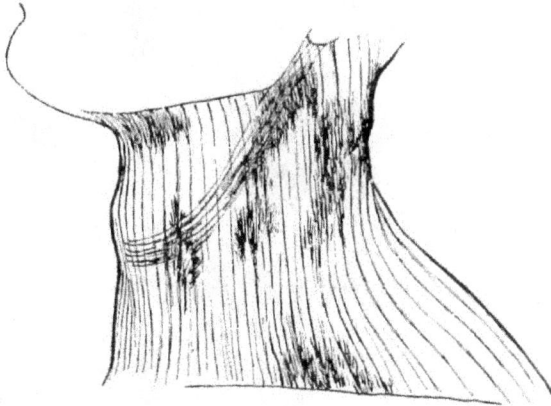

Fig. 6b.

Affections of the head and neck.

Adhesions in the neck preventing the normal glandular secretion. Adhesions in the upper part of the throat causing laryngitis. Adhesions at the back of the neck preventing normal circulation *via* lymphatic ganglia. Adhesions preventing normal flow of current to lungs.

of the human body, to the problem of illness, or disorder in the human mechanism.

It may be stated as a general rule that all illnesses are caused through some kind of disorder in the flow of nervous current. Such disorders are generally caused by adhesions of the muscular fibres. These adhesions may arise suddenly through an accident (such as crushing by a heavy object) or gradually, through constant exercise of a single part of the body, or through exposure to draughts or damp, causing the skin to adhere to the muscles. Such adhesions, though slight at first, obstruct the passage of the nervous current; the adhesion consequently becomes more obstinate, until finally the passage of the nervous current becomes completely blocked, the tissues fail to be reproduced, and the organ in question loses its suppleness. This condition is an important basis of disease.

The whole question of ill-health presents itself simply enough: how is it possible for a man who has never studied or even taken any real notice of his own body, its powers and functions and needs, to keep this machine of his in good working order?

When anything goes wrong, he feels a pain, and says that such-and- such a place is hurting, or that he feels tired or ill; but he knows neither the cause nor the remedy. He performs his daily actions mechanically, standing in the same position for long periods, fatiguing and hardening the joints of the legs, or sitting hunched up in a chair, so that the circulation in the legs is diminished, whilst the curvature of the spine arrests the flow of the nervous currents which are consequently insufficiently distributed to the abdomen and lower limbs. When he thinks or writes or reads with his head bowed, the circulation of the blood in the head becomes irregular and breathing is restricted. In general, whether at work or at play, he exercises the right side more than the left, developing one part more than the other. He destroys the equilibrium of the body similarly when he sleeps with his head on too many pillows, when he eats too quickly foods which are irritating or indigestible to his stomach (which he feeds twice or thrice as much as it needs), or again when he drinks alcoholic and other harmful drinks when he is not thirsty anyway.

All these habits put the human machine out of order and create those disorders of the mind, the nerves and the blood which are commonly called illnesses.

We will not go into further detail as to the cause of ill-health, for the essential facts are simple enough, and the world in general has no time for books which are not amusing. We will only say that man desires pleasure and amusement, which he enjoys through the medium of his senses, his mind and his spirit, yet the poor fellow refuses to take any account of the very instrument by which he enjoys these pleasures. Humanity in general neither walks, eats, sleeps nor talks normally. Man's whole appearance and way of living is disordered.

All we ask is that man shall acquire an understanding and conscious knowledge of his visible and invisible self, so that he may live as human beings should live.

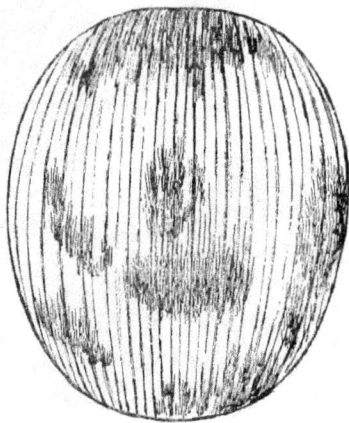

Fig. 6c.

Affections at the source of energy.
Adhesions of cranial nerves causing
diminished supply of the ultra-sensitive
vibrations to pineal gland.
Adhesions causing mental and psychotic
disorders.

CHAPTER VI
HOW WE SHOULD BE CURED

AS we have already explained, the human machine is made up of various kinds of fibres, the fibres of the bones, the muscles, the tendons and the nerves. If these fibres fail to receive a sufficient supply of nervous current they stick together, forming what are known as adhesions. The removal of these adhesions is the essential process in the cure of all disease.

A study of the formation of adhesions in muscular and nerve-fibres, together with an adequate description of their consequences and the mode of their removal, would occupy a volume in itself All we can give here is a brief general indication of the way in which adhesions can be eliminated.

How adhesions are Removed

The procedure may be divided into two parts: preparation and manipulation. Just as the artist's clay must be prepared for the modelling, so the affected part must be prepared by rubbing with oil (preferably oil of almonds), to render the muscles as supple and pliable as possible. This facilitates the manipulative part — the separation of the tissues with the fingers.

First, by a transverse or "horizontal " movement of the fingers the skin must be separated from the underlying muscle. Then the muscular fibres themselves must be separated vertically with a degree of pressure conformable to their condition. If too much force is employed there is a risk of breaking through the protecting sheaths covering the fibres, which would cause pain. But if too little pressure is exerted the fibres will not separate. Hence the need for highly sensitive fingers able to distinguish between thick and thin fibres, etc.

After long experience and practice the fingers are able to feel the exact condition of the tissues. Sometimes for instance, the bones of the joints seem to be swollen: actually this is an indication of the hardening of the surrounding muscle. In such cases the fingers must work with great precaution for the fibres are very dried up and may snap in the attempt to separate them.

But it must be clearly understood that the mastery of these methods is no easy task, and should not be undertaken without the supervision of an experienced pranotherapist, able to give advice as to individual treatment and to prevent over-exertion. Pranotherapy entails no blind manipulation; it requires a highly developed consciousness and sensitivity, attained only by hours of patient daily practice on the living body.

The Order of Removal of Adhesions

Long years of practice have convinced us of our theory that treatment must begin in the head, with the adjustment of the cranial muscles. That is to say, all the muscular fibres must be separated and put in place, and it must be seen that the skin does not adhere in any way, so that the maximum number of currents required by a healthy organism is given free access to the body.

Then the medulla oblongata must be freed from all kinds of adherence to allow these accumulated and condensed currents to be distributed throughout the whole body. Next the whole base of the cranium must

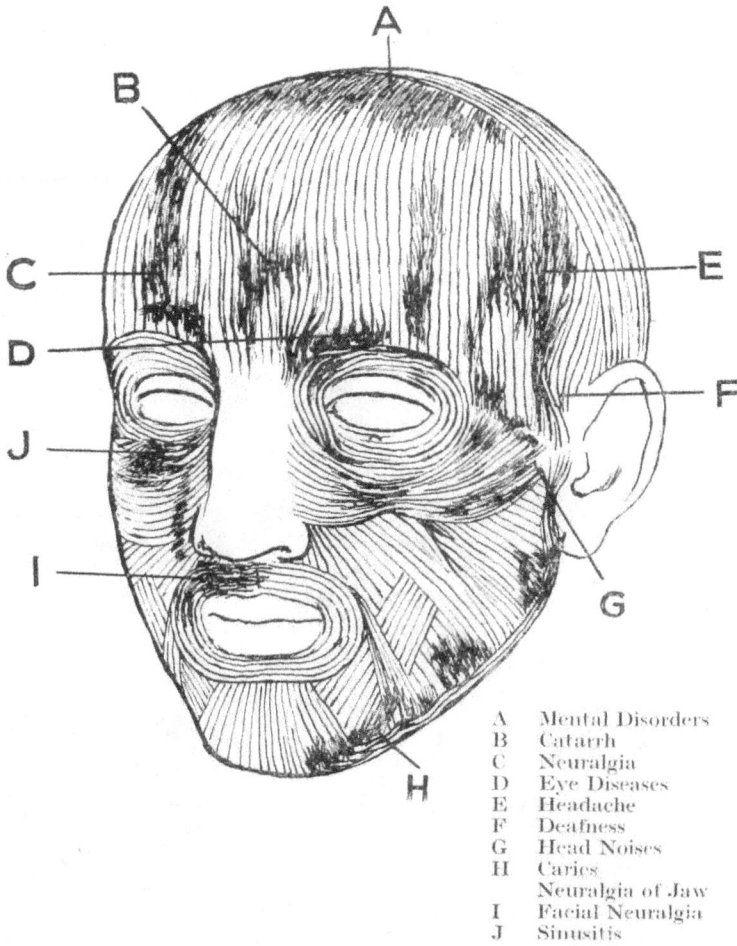

A	Mental Disorders
B	Catarrh
C	Neuralgia
D	Eye Diseases
E	Headache
F	Deafness
G	Head Noises
H	Caries
	Neuralgia of Jaw
I	Facial Neuralgia
J	Sinusitis

Fig. 7a.

Indicating the different forms of disease caused
by adhesions in different parts of the body. The
adhesions prevent the passage of the nervous
current. with the result that the organs are insufficiently nourished and the function badly.   (See
Chapter V)   (Head)

be disengaged, giving access to the two holes in the spinal column on either side of the Atlas, in order that the sensitive fibres may supply nervous current to the sympathetic ganglia.

All the neck muscles beside the cervical vertebra, the muscles and Nerve fibres of the forehead (controlling mental disorders), all the various openings in the head (eyes, ears, nostrils, mouth), the frontal and maxillary sinuses and the joints of the jaw-bones must be thoroughly in trim to assist the functioning of all the senses.

The muscles of the eyes must be released and the nerve fibres set in position, so that the whole form of the eyes is restored to normality. By this means short sight, long sight, astigmatism, etc, are done away with.

By the elimination of all adhesions in the throat, the pharyngeal plexus[1] is restored to its normal functions. This plexus, which has sixteen branches, feeds all the glands below the jaw and passes on the nervous current in three main streams; two to the lungs and the third to the sternum and bronchial tubes, the heart (the cardiac plexus) and the solar plexus at the base of the sternum, which controls the movements of the diaphragm during respiration.

Next comes the adjustment of all the muscles of the thorax to free all the nerve fibres and nerve centres which help the thorax to perform the bellows-like action of normal breathing. When breathing is completely normal and absolutely unrestricted there can be no disease of the lungs or any other part of the body.

1 Sanskrit *canth-chakr*e or throat—plexus

The lumbar muscles must next be restored to normal to allow the lumbar plexus to supply nervous current to the intestines. All the abdominal muscles must be freed and the nervous current restored from the diaphragm to the pelvis to promote the normal functioning of the liver, the bile vesicles, the pancreas, the stomach, the spleen, the intestines, the kidneys, the bladder and the genital organs. In this way all kinds of male and female weaknesses may be cured.

Both edges of the hips must be completely freed from muscular adhesions to allow of a free and regular distribution of currents to the sciatic and other nerve fibres of the legs.

All the leg muscles must be readjusted to assume their normal form with the maximum circulation of blood and nervous current, and the knees, ankles and the various joints of the feet must be cleared of small adhesions. In the same way the shoulder blades, the collar-bone, the elbows, the wrists, the joints of the hands and all the muscles of the arm must be entirely free to allow the circulation of the blood and the nervous current to go on reproducing fresh tissues to replace those which are worn out or dried up through illness. By this means, and in conjunction with a properly arranged diet, arthritis, rheumatism, all kinds of neuritis, etc. can be eliminated.

On the other side of the body all the vertebra (cervical, dorsal, lumbar, sacral and coccygeal) must be freed of all adhesions, and the thirty three vertebra separated, put in position and rendered supple like those of a serpent.

The distribution of the nervous currents must meet with no obstruction of any kind, As they leave the medulla oblongata the currents must be able to pass freely and in due proportion throughout the whole body.

Pranotherapy

To the method of treatment which we have just outlined we have given the name of *Pranotherapy*. (*Prana* has been described in previous chapters — *therapy*, method of cure.) By this method we repair the human machine and regenerate the entire body. But a Pranotherapist capable of regenerating a whole organism must first of all have made an anatomical study of the living body, particularly his own, and have restored normal functioning power to every part of his body. For if the Pranotherapist is not familiar with the normal state of every organ, joint, muscle and fibre, he cannot diagnose their abnormal states. Secondly, the Pranotherapist must never ask the patient what is wrong; he must find out himself; and by explaining the precise nature of the malady, will increase the patient's confidence in him. To be capable of this the Pranotherapist must develop his sensitive faculties to such a degree that he can feel the currents of the human body from the top of the head to the tips of the toes and ascertain the condition of the circulation of nervous vibrations. He must be able to find out the spot at which the currents have been arrested. He must be able to adjust his treatment to the strength of the patient, for if he exerts too much pressure he will do harm, and if he exerts insufficient pressure he will do nothing at all.

The teaching of Pranotherapy is even more difficult than the practice of the Pranotherapist, for the teacher must have practical experience of all that he talks about, and must be able to answer questions on physical, nervous, mental, spiritual and moral matters.

The *physical education* needed by man would provide him with a body neither fat nor thin, tense or flabby, but proportionate, strong and supple.

The movements of our method are linked with the Hatha Yoga, the system evolved by the Indian Yogis for the maintenance of muscular equilibrium. They begin with the toes and end at the head, exercising to the full the stretching power of all the muscles and the flexibility of all the joints, so that every limb is developed in the appropriate way.

The object of these purely physical exercises is the restoration of the normal circulation of the blood and the separation of all the muscular fibres, to prevent the formation of adhesions which are the cause of muscular and nervous ailments, All this prepares the way for *nervous education,*[1] a system of exercises combining slow movements of the limbs with the three forms of breathing (abdominal, thoracic and mental), This combination is a powerful aid to the attainment of mental equilibrium, perfect health and prolonged youth.

Physical Exercises

The scope of this book does not permit of a detailed list of physical exercises, and therefore we propose to publish, later, a complete manual of physical culture. Here we confine ourselves to a brief but representative

---

1 See our forthcoming publication: Self-Mastery through the Control of the Nervous System,

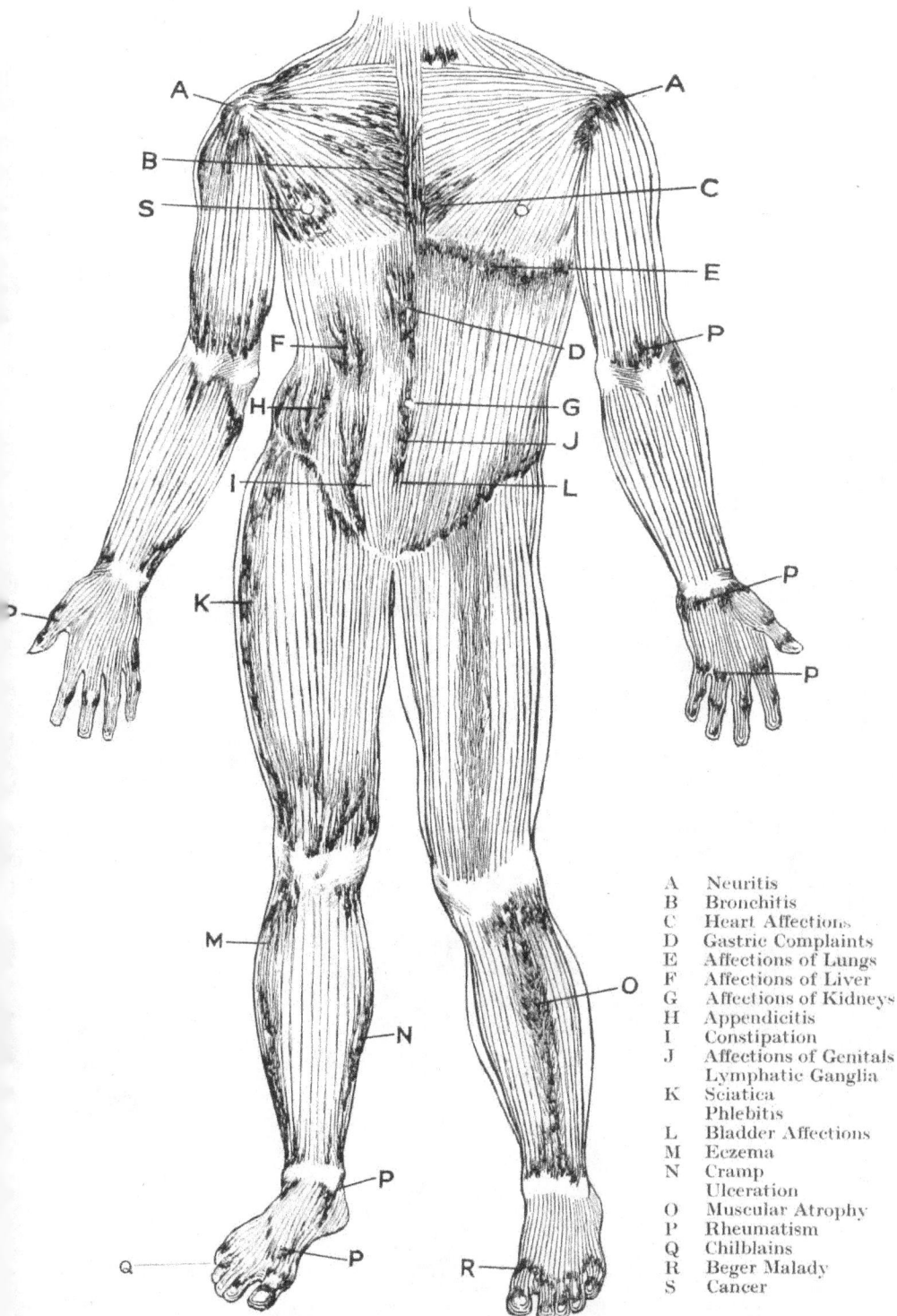

A	Neuritis
B	Bronchitis
C	Heart Affections
D	Gastric Complaints
E	Affections of Lungs
F	Affections of Liver
G	Affections of Kidneys
H	Appendicitis
I	Constipation
J	Affections of Genitals
	Lymphatic Ganglia
K	Sciatica
	Phlebitis
L	Bladder Affections
M	Eczema
N	Cramp
	Ulceration
O	Muscular Atrophy
P	Rheumatism
Q	Chilblains
R	Beger Malady
S	Cancer

Fig 7b.   As Fig. 7a (Front)

selection of exercises which will serve as examples of the best method of develop-ing the different parts of the body, beginning with the feet and ending with the head.

All the following exercises are performed lying down, to the accompaniment of deep breathing and of thorough relaxation between movements.

Feet, Ankles and Legs

Lie flat on the back and exercise all the muscles of the toes and feet by alternately contracting and relaxing them in every possible direction. Then move the feet round and back in a slow rotatory rhythm; this makes the ankle muscles supple. Next draw the toes forward and back, feeling the leg muscles alternately contract and relax.

Abdomen, Spine, Arms and Legs

Next bend the knees and raise them as high as possible towards the abdomen. Then lower them as slowly as possible, breathing steadily and deeply. At least ten breaths should be taken before the feet reach the floor.

Raise the arms above the head until they are resting on the floor, palms upward. At the same time contract the muscles of the fingers and toes, breathing deeply. Still breathing deeply, raise the left arm and leg until the foot can be grasped by the hand, the leg being kept absolutely stiff Contract the muscles of the whole body, then slowly lower the arm and leg to their original positions. Repeat with the right arm and leg.

From their position (on the floor above the head, palms upward) raise both arms until they are at right-angles to the body, contract the muscles of the hands (fingers spread) and lower the arms slowly, first towards the head, then towards the body. Return to the original position.

Raise both legs (knees stiff) until they form a right-angle with the body. Lower them as slowly as possible, breathing deeply.

Raise the trunk slowly until it is at right-angles to the legs; lower slowly.

Spine

Lie with head and soles of feet resting on the floor supporting the rest of the body; the arms bent at the elbow, palms touching, fingers spread, thumbs on chest. Contract the muscles of the whole body and slowly lower it until the last (coccygeal) bone of the spine is touching the floor.

Thorax

Lie face downwards, hands clasped behind the back. Perform a "rolling" movement by resting the weight of the body alternately on one shoulder and on the other. Return to the first position and perform a "rocking" movement by contracting the muscles from the diaphragm to the clavicle and alternately raising and lowering this part of the body.

Pelvis, Sternum and Spine

Lie on the back, arms to sides, and contract the muscles of the legs and feet (toes forward). Then (keeping both knees stiff) extend first one leg, then the next, feeling the pelvic muscles work as alternate hips are pulled downward. Raise the arms above the head and repeat the exercise with the arms instead of the legs. Then perform both movements together, extending left leg simultaneously with right arm, and vice versa.

This is a most valuable exercise for counteracting adhesions in the muscular fibres of the spine, sternum and pelvis.

Thorax and Back

Lie on the back, hands by sides, palms up. Move the arms slowly round to the head, describing a semi-circle with each arm. Return slowly.

Neck

Lie on the back, arms out at right-angles on the floor, palms up, Raise the head slowly and try to touch the chest with the chin, but without moving the shoulders. Lower slowly. Raise the head again and turn to the left; lower slowly in this position. Repeat, turning to the right.

Breathing

We have studied the different kinds of breathing advocated by the science of Yoga, which expounds the theory of the Pranayama, or regularising of the vital (Pranic) currents, This exercise, we find, has two parts, assimilative and distributive; the assimilation of the vital currents is achieved through meditation, and their distribution and regularisation is achieved through breathing.

There are various methods of cultivating meditation and breathing, but before dealing with these we must mention their necessary pre-conditions. If the respiratory apparatus (for breathing) and the cerebral apparatus (for meditation) are not in a properly functioning state, how will it be possible to obtain satisfactory results ?

Here are the essential requirements of proper breathing: all the joints of the spine and sternum must be absolutely flexible; if the pectoral, dorsal and intercostal muscles have become hardened or shrunken so that they cannot contract freely, how will it be possible for the lungs to open up completely in an easy and natural expansion'? And if breathing is forced, the muscular tissues are reproduced excessively, the thorax stiffens and the lungs press down on the heart, which begins to suffer from over-exertion. Breathing in these circumstances does harm rather than good.

We must pass on to the conditions for effective meditation: if the muscles of the neck, forehead and head are not supple they will be incapable of thorough relaxation. Meditation in such circumstances is impossible and, if induced forcibly, is liable to derange the mind. We have known of students of Yoga who have lost their reason through attempting advanced mental breathing when in an unfit state; we have even heard of cases in which the skull was burst open through the electrical force generated by excessively violent mental exertion.

To avoid all these dangers the student must have his general condition examined and perfected by a practising pranotherapist who can give him practical instruction as to how to restore to their normal state all the joints, muscles and nerves of his body before he begins these exercises of respiration and meditation.

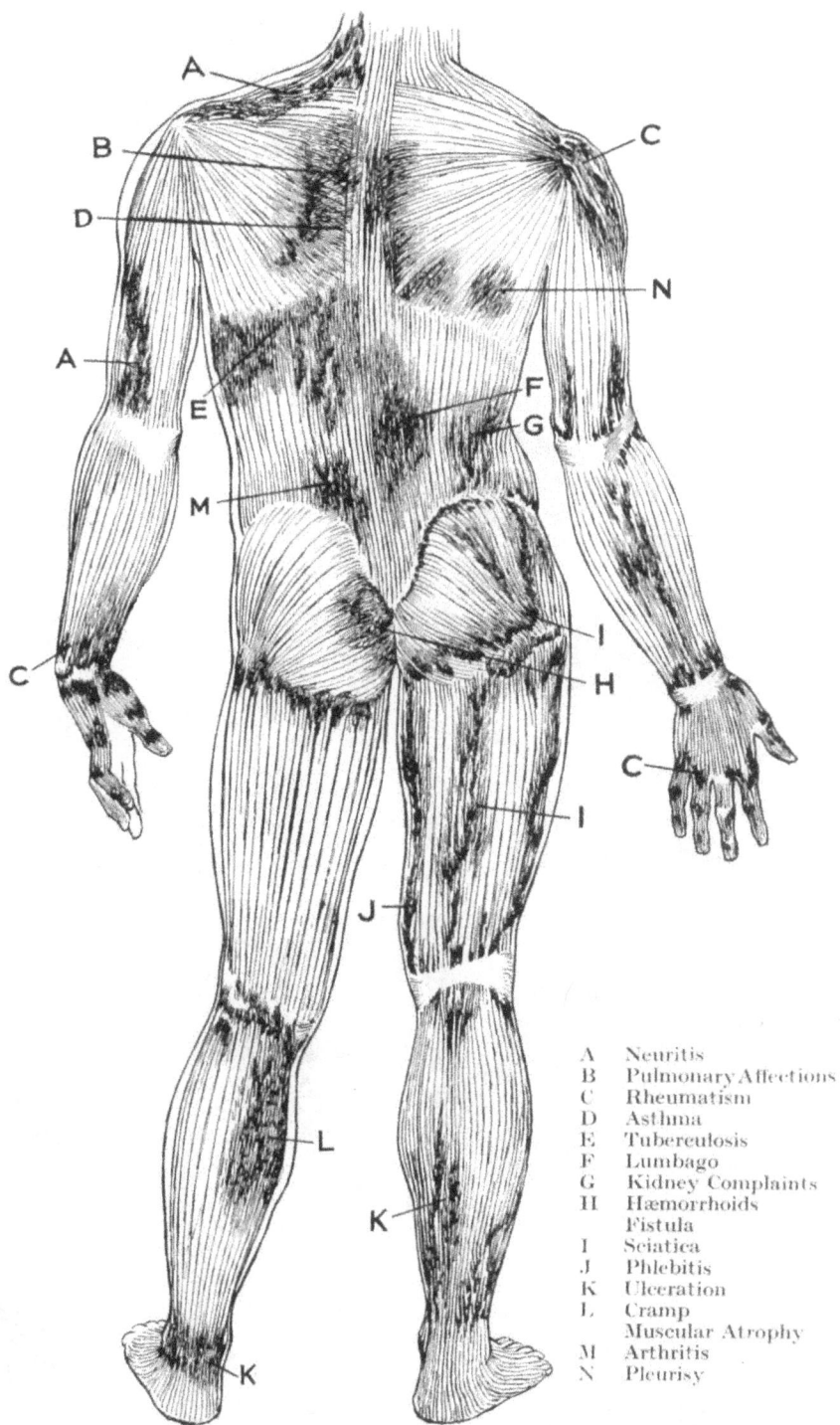

A	Neuritis
B	Pulmonary Affections
C	Rheumatism
D	Asthma
E	Tuberculosis
F	Lumbago
G	Kidney Complaints
H	Hæmorrhoids
	Fistula
I	Sciatica
J	Phlebitis
K	Ulceration
L	Cramp
	Muscular Atrophy
M	Arthritis
N	Pleurisy

Fig 7c. As Fig. 7a (Back)

When he is in a fit condition to perform them, the student may start with the following exercises.

Exercise 1 — Mental breathing: Lie on the back, knees bent, soles of the feet touching, left hand on the neck. Place the two middle fingers of the right hand on the left nostril, the index finger on the forehead between the eyebrows, and the thumb on the right nostril, Now raise the thumb and breathe in up the right nostril, slowly and deeply so that the air passes along the cartilage in the centre of the nose, avoiding the membrane on the outer side. Breathe as deeply as possible, concentrating the thoughts on the upward. movement of the air. Then breathe out slowly, this time concentrating the thoughts on the pranic currents which are now flowing downward towards the feet.

This exercise must be performed three times with the same nostril — twice as explained above, and the third time in the following way: after breathing in, replace the thumb to stop all respiration, and fix the attention (eyes shut) on the index finger between the eyebrows. Then remove the two middle fingers covering the left nostril, and breathe out on this side.

Now repeat the whole exercise starting with the left nostril, so that the final expiration is on the right side.

The complete exercise should be performed three times at first, then one additional time until the end of the week; after this continue without further increases for a month.

Exercise II — Thoracic breathing: Lie on the back with the legs together, hands against thighs, body completely relaxed. Take in a deep breath; now concentrate the attention on a point in the centre of the diaphragm, and imagine the air passing from here to the middle of the breast-bone and upward to the cartilage between the two nostrils and on to the middle of the cranium; then feel it pass down the spinal column to the coccyx, and rise again through the middle of the abdomen to the point of departure in the diaphragm. Breathe out. Repeat this at least seven times. This exercise opens up the nerve centres.

Exercise III — Abdominal breathing: Lie as for the previous exercise. Take a deep breath; dilating the abdomen and feeling the contraction of the muscles from the groin to the clavicle. In this position hold the breath for at least ten seconds, then breathe out slowly until the abdomen is so deflated that a slight contraction of the lumbar muscles is felt. Repeat at least seven times. This exercise regularises the functioning of the digestive tract and all the abdominal organs; it also ensures the normal flow of currents to the arms and legs.

All three exercises must be performed after a thorough emptying of the bowels and bladder. They should never be undertaken directly after meals. The best time for them is the morning, preferably the early morning. At first they will seem difficult, but after performing them daily for some time the student will gain mastery of them, and derive from them confidence, courage, energy and the firm desire to persevere until he has complete control over his muscular, nervous and mental activity, and is able to direct all his actions whether seen or unseen in the full understanding of life and the complete fulfillment of his social duty.

Chapter VII
THE RESULTS OF OUR METHOD

IN the course of twenty two years we have cured all kinds of different ailments, some of our cases having been declared incurable by the medical world. First, we must mention the various sorts of paralysis: infantile paralysis, hemiplegia, paraplegia, Little's disease, Parkinson's disease (paralysis agitans), disseminated sclerosis, and facial paralysis have responded favourably to our treatment, even long-standing cases of twenty years old, in which the limbs had lost all trace of sensibility.

Then we have treated cases of neurasthenia, loss of memory, migraine, headaches; all kinds of adhesions, neuritis, arthritis, etc.; tuberculosis of the lungs, intestines and joints, gastric troubles, disorders of the liver and intestines, duodenal and other ulcers, varicoceles; even cancer in its first stages, and atrophy of the limbs have been cured by pranotherapy.

We have obtained good results in combating sexual impotence, even in cases where all sexual desire was extinct. We have also successfully treated fibroids, prostatitis, and inflammation of the matrix.

Next we must cite cases of myopia, presbyopia, astigmatism and deafness. But we cannot give the names of all the ailments we have successfully treated — we can only say that further testimony of our results can be supplied by qualified doctors and professors. So far, we have cured 338 doctors of medicine of various nationalities. We have documents to prove this, which are at the disposal of any medical authority which may desire to see them.

Individual Cases

It may be of interest to cite a few typical examples of cases of chronic disorder which have been cured by pranotherapy.

In 1923 we treated a case of poliomyelitis (an infection of the spinal cord which causes paralysis) of eleven years' standing, The patient came to us in a bath chair, both legs being completely atrophied. He had been all over the Continent visiting neurologists and specialists of various kinds, all of whom had condemned him to the life of a cripple. After a few months' treatment by pranotherapy he was able to walk,

This recalls another case of infantile paralysis dating from 1918. The patient came to us in 1929, his legs so atrophied that he was unable to stand. Now he can climb four flights of stairs unaided.

A girl of twenty suffering from tuberculosis was declared by her doctors to have another fortnight to live. Her weight was under six stones; she was unable to eat; her kidneys and bladder had ceased to function; her temperature would not drop below 104. After pranotherapeutic treatment she was completely cured. She has now almost doubled her weight, is married and has a healthy child.

Another of our patients was a lady dress designer whose deafness obliged her to use an acoustic apparatus. After thirty days of our treatment, one of her customers, the wife of a well-known doctor, expressed her surprise at being able to carry on a conversation without the aid of the apparatus, The "deaf" lady replied that she had thrown the apparatus into the dustbin, since she was now able to hear naturally. This so impressed the doctor's wife that she sent her husband to us to be treated for his deafness, which also was successfully cured.

An English colonel fell from his horse in 1916 during the Great War, with the result that his brain ceased to function; he could not even cross the road alone. He came to us in 1930 and was cured by pranotherapy in two months.

We have treated successfully literally hundreds of cases of dilatation of the stomach. The general method of treatment in each case was to restore the nervous equilibrium by loosening the muscles below the diaphragm, the contraction of which was causing the atrophy of the pylorus. This ensured normal reproduction of tissues and automatic con- traction and relaxation of the stomach-muscles, which in turn induced the return of normal digestion and assimilation,

Conditions of Cure

1. *Age of Patient.* Children are cured more quickly than old people, whose tissues are created more slowly and who must consequently be more patient in the expectation of complete cure.

2. *State of Disorder.* If the disorder is recent, it is quickly cured; if it has been going on for years, the dried-up or malformed tissues must first be eradicated, the flow of blood and nervous current must first then be restored to provide fresh tissues and so restore the normal functioning of the organs. This naturally takes longer.

3. *Temperature.* If the atmosphere is warm, the circulation is active and the tissues are quickly formed; if it is cold the formation of tissues slows down. The same is true of plants, which grow quickly in hot weather.

Individual Treatment

Although we have treated more than twenty thousand patients, we have never seen two cases alike. This is in conformity with the law of Nature that identicals do not exist. We have met with some two thousand cases of stomach trouble, but never two of precisely the same kind. What is known as heart trouble may be traced to innumerable different causes: sometimes the cardiac plexus is obstructed in some way, another time there is a large adhesion pressing on the aorta below the diaphragm and preventing the regular movement of the heart; or again we have seen loss of movement, of the ribs caused by the drying-up of the intercostal muscles, leading to a diminution of breathing power and thence to the restriction and malformation of the heart.

We have treated various cases of intermittent beating of the heart, In demonstrations before several doctors we have lowered the pulsation of the blood from one hundred to seventy. We have also cured cases in which the patient felt continual pain after a completed operation, as the result of some adhesion caused by the surgical treatment,

Thus it may be seen that the basis of pranotherapy is individual treatment; it makes no generalisation of illnesses, lt is a unique method, but after practising it. for the last twenty two years we feel justified in making known its positive results.

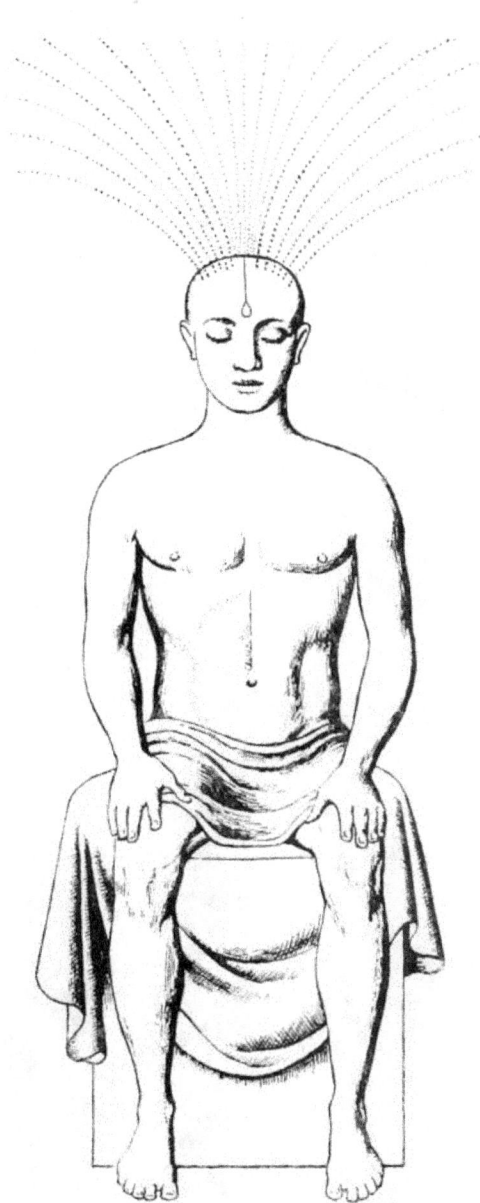

The pose for the voluntary assimilation
of additional sensitive and ultra-sensitive
currents from the atmosphere. The body
must be completely relaxed, all though
concentrated on the pineal glad receiving
the cosmic vibrations

Connective Tissue

"The connective tissue, in short, is like the all pervading ether in the physical universe"
— Initis Dr Andrea Rabagliati 1916

Since the first International Fascia Research Congress was held at Harvard Medical School, Boston in 2007 there has been something of an explosion of interest and research into the connective tissue and fascia. Yet, as the opening quote above and the quotes below demonstrate, the function of connective tissue and fascia has been of vital interest to practitioners from the earliest days of manual therapy.

"The fascia gives one of, if not the greatest problems to solve as to the part it takes in life and death. It belts each muscle, vein, nerve, and all organs of the body. It is almost a network of nerves, cells and tubes, running to and from it; it is crossed and filled with, no doubt, millions of nerve centers and fibers to carry on the work of secreting and excreting fluid vital and destructive. By its action we live, and by its failure we shrink, or swell, and die."

"the soul of a man with all the streams of pure living water seems to dwell in the fascia of the body."
— The Philosophy of Osteopathy A.T. Still 1899

Robert Hall MD who met and watched Stone working in 1970 in India reported that when treating patients Stone would look for and release 'connective tissue locks.'

"He pressed on pressure points, taught exercises, advised diet changes, and ran his powerful hands over the body, stopping always in specific places to release what he called connective tissue locks."

47

" We need to get the currents flowing. Energy locks. It's a gas problem."

— Robert Hall 1993

In Stone's teaching career between 1950 and 1973 he often came back to the concept of 'connective tissue locks,' yet his written books on Polarity Therapy have relatively few references to the connective tissue and fascia of the body. Nevertheless a focus on connective tissue formed an extensive part of his teaching. In a seminar given in August 1972 Stone said:

"The connective tissue is the conveyer. The secret of the conveyor of the lymph and the prana energy through the collagen fibres. And when you have tendons like these naturally when you stretch them out you are pulling on the connective tissue sheath so the gas inside there in the collagen fibre can move and let the current through.

As soon it does the pain is gone, the pain is pressure - like the pressure against a dam that wants to blow the dam up and the water get carried away......... And this phenomenon can't be explained in any other way. Why? Nobody has given any attention to the connective tissues and it is because we have not taken into consideration this overall turnover of the five pranas and the five tattvas, this radiating energy that we can't help but to receive...but it's there...but you can refuse it, you can shut it out and if you can get mad enough you can't always stop yourself from hauling off and hitting something. In other words its expression, a natural action and reaction of these five energies and they are in the hands and they are in the toes. And you say "Oh, Nonsense, I pulled toes before," there isn't hardly anybody in the field that hasn't pulled toes sometime or at least the leg of someone.(audience laughter)...... Don't forget that when I get the idea across.

I can't tell you how to pull anybody's leg but I can tell you how to pull a toe that will get results that will astonish you. And it is because of that that I am going into this fundamental thing that it is the electromagnetic energy as a gas that gets locked, as a plasma gas and when you straighten this out and put your finger where the lock is, as a fulcrum and then we straighten it either by flexion or by extension, you are moving the collagen fibre block as a gas, and that's the mystery and why the connective tissue? Because the connective tissue moves the bones. Your muscles do not move the bones directly – you see they always end up in a tendon. These are all flexors or extensors.

The condensation of the circulatory, the contraction of the circulation that furnishes the blood supply to the muscles by which it bulges laterally in the belly and shortens the two ends, ends at the tendons. Then tendon has to convey that impulse but if that tendon is contracted by a tension field and the electromagnetic force of the plasma is not moving, the prana can't go through because the gas is a block. That gas is sedimentation. It is an emotional lock. That's why emotions can raise such heck. That's why I give you this simple energy stretch so that you can do something for yourself instead of reaching into the cabinet for something. Just get quiet enough and go back into the mother's space womb and there you find the answer." [1]

It is apparent from his final lectures that Stone did not think that there is actually plasma gas in the tissues as such, particularly since he was only aware of the extremely hot gas plasmas rather than the more recent discoveries of cold i.e. room temperature plasmas. He related the plasma gas to the emotional energy of mind. In 1973 he said that our emotions are similar to this plasma gas:

"They put us through all these contortions, we go through all these emotions, heat and temperature, miseries mental and emotional, not the heat of millions of degrees though."

To a large degree this usage of a modern scientific metaphor obscures the true depth of the energy model that Stone was actually working with. When talking about the movement capacities of the human body and the connective tissue structure, the energy that Stone was referring to was, rather than being plasma gas or simple life energy, in fact, the energetic emanations from the heart or air chakra and the related air element or airy principle. This airy activity in the human being is also referred to in India as the subtle or vital airs. In Ayurvedic teaching these are the five vayu being; prana vayu, udana vayu, samana vayu, vyana vayu and apana vayu.

The word vayu translates as "wind," and the root 'va' means "that which flows" – and so a vayu is a "vital force" that moves throughout the body controlling functions such as digestion, respiration and nervous impulses as well as the consciousness that lies behind those impulses.

All of the five prana vayu have an influence on physical movement in various ways. However, the most significant of these in relation to connective tissue is vyana vayu being the watery aspect of the air energy and samana vayu which is related to the fiery aspect of this airy energy.

Vyana moves from the core out to the periphery.

Samana moves from the periphery of the body into the core.

This movement of energy from the core out to the periphery and from the periphery to the core is intrinsic to the Polarity theory and relates to the fundamental energetic pulsation of centrifugal and centripetal movement.

Vyana Vayu – translates as 'outward moving air.' It moves throughout the whole body. Vyana governs the functions of the muscles, joints, nerves and veins as well circulating physical nutrients and the life force. Its function is binding or cohesive. It manifests as the 'surface tension' of our energy and physical bodies. Vyana also functions through sensory awareness and is

50

essential to our experience of 'self' as an integrated whole and gives rise to our sense of boundaries both physically and emotionally. In a general sense it controls the functioning of all the muscles, and is experienced in the skin.

Samana Vayu – translates as 'the balancing air.' In a physical sense it governs the metabolism or 'fire of digestion' as it is referred to in Polarity Therapy and the functioning of the digestive organs and glands. It governs our powers of discrimination and discernment granting us the ability to judge that which is helpful or harmful to us. It is also our 'will' and relates to our voluntary engagement with the world in terms of movement and relating to others.

The samana is linked to the thought processes behind voluntary controls that activate the musculature to move us towards or away from certain experiences and the vyana is the energy that controls the physical functioning of the various connective tissues.

In his later work Stone had a strong focus on the activity of the air element in the human being largely due to its role in the elimination of wastes and the fact that it governs the overall movement of all the energies within the human energy system.

"They tell us that the ancients used to say that man dies because his kidneys do not function. The kidneys are the Libra, the airy principle, the shoulders and down to here (the ankles), the airy principle. That is the solar energy that goes around and when that solar energy can't go down and the gas, or the plasma cannot be separated or go into the water principle and be separated by the kidneys then you have swelling and stagnant conditions and what not because it this heel - this is the scales Libra right here."

Stone – Seminar August 1972

He focused specifically on manipulation of the negative pole of the air element in the body which is in the Achilles tendon.

"And in the tendon Achilles there lies the big story. Achilles was one of the great warriors of the city of Troy and nobody could overcome him, the tendon of Achilli is an outstanding phenomena. [These things have a way of disappearing when you want something. Looking for an illustration] This gives a good view of the side. I show you that and the tendon Achilli is cut off here. This is not the one I wanted to show you. I have a better one than that. There it is, all at once it came back!, now the gastrocnemius muscle has two belly lines here on the side and there is the reflex on the abdomen and the soleus, here the soleus is peeled back underneath and there's another one along side of it gracilis, soleus and plantaris, it's the smaller one that goes along side but these tendons, see how much sheath of the tendon you have here and when you cut this you are literally cutting the conduction to the heel where everything is settled. The heel is the furthest and the densest and the most direct physical contact if you step on the toes so you don't get the shock from the heels. Everything condenses in the heels..................What they are really meaning to say is the condensation of the vital energy passing through this heavy tendon, which it must pass through in order to get the major energy back that why it is so disadvantageous to wear rubber soles because it does not ground us enough and there is too much accumulation of waste products or magnetism which hinders the circulation in the collagen fibres. This a major and when we get to work on it, when you lay the patient down and you work on it with the flat of the hand and you work out all this tension of the tendon Achilles you find it is so sore here it is almost impossible to touch. And that's that gas in there. And if I didn't tell you what it was you would think it was your compression massage that was the miracle. The miracle is to understand what you're moving, you are moving this gas in the tendon and the fibres of the tendons which are hollow, the collagen fibres. And when you do this static gas which is the bulk of the Universe which is everywhere, then the current can go through and the release is so instant that you can correlate it with all the other functions of the body and

the five senses. When you cut this and this does not take place then you are really lost.

But what I am trying to say is that the five energies which are locked up in the movement of the prana through the tension fields can be moved here and unblocked. In other words, by this manipulation when you come to the two muscles here which are two belly muscles, the soleus and the gastrocnemius you pinch them together and find a great deal of pressure and you can use this for leverage. You can use flexion and extension and at the same time deep pressure here and you will release all this."

"And it's the energy - the prana in the sun that makes this level and this filter possible. So when you work on this and work out this tension here you are working on the major and your are using it with leverage of flexion and with leverage of extension but the pressure is always against the tension here on the tendon upward and on the sides here to bring them together....and here when you get on the hallucis longus on the outside here and the digitorum there you would think it was the tendon but no it was the lock of the airy principle of the prana, of the scales of the sulphur energy that is locked there not in the tendon as soon as the gas moves this tendon is the thing with every other tendon only it happens to be there and usually here you find the kernel and it can be right in the bone it does not have to be in the tendon but it is usually so close around the tendon and the first time I gave the demonstration we pushed this through the liver by flipping this it was very painful but it got results, you could relax the tension of torticollis in about half an hour or twenty minutes by releasing tension fields and that is what you have to understand otherwise you think this thing has no physical foundation. I will show you that the gas may be anywhere in the bones, in the articulations of the talus anywhere along in here, you can find the soreness right in the bones anywhere one of them, the cuboid, remember Dr Locke he adjusted the cuboid of a man that advertised (for help) he was so busy the rest of his life adjusting the cuboid, this is the cuboid bone because you move the gas that happens to let go the tension in the ring and this gas tension you can find it anywhere but you have got to be able to detect it."

Stone – Seminar August 1972

The technique Stone is referring to in this lecture is show below in figure 2.

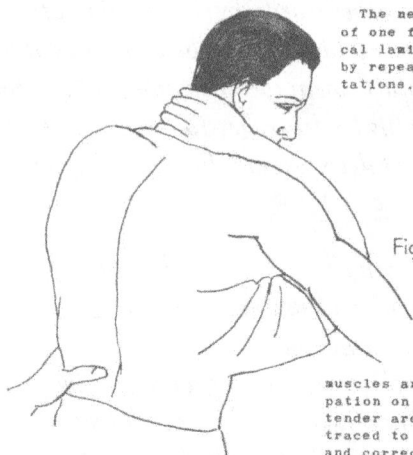

The neck contact requires the pressure of one finger specifically on one cervical lamina, to release the impulse there by repeated stretching movements and rotations.

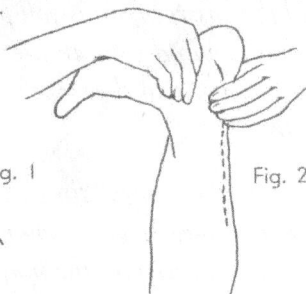

Fig. 1   Fig. 2

The neck is the positive pole to the negative lumbar region. This Polarity relationship is illustrated in VITALITY BALANCE page 15, chart 2. Stimulation above and adjustments below are carried on simultaneously. The direction of the thumb fulcrum determines the specific adjustment to be made. See "Country-side Technique" in WIRELESS ANATOMY, pages 54-59. This specific contact with leverage is the quickest correction for all lumbar inferior and posterior subluxations; also for lateral side slips. It is unique for Sciatica and leg conditions.

Cervicals and lumbars are opposites on the double 'S' curve of the spine, and in direct line of leverage by the spinal

muscles and gravity pull. By careful palpation on the cervical laminae, the most tender area can be found on one side and traced to the corresponding lumbar lesion, and corrected.

Have the patient sit well back on a stool. Place your arm under the shoulder, on the side where you found the sorest cervical, and swing the posterior side anteriorly. The arm should fit snugly under the shoulder and the hand below the occiput, over the atlas, for a 5th L. posterior; on the axis for a 4th, etc.

If the sympathetic and parasympathetic have been released first, the adjustment will happen naturally by correct position and the leverage used.

Fig. 2 - The foot is leveraged on the leg and released repeatedly with one hand while the other hand works out the energy blocks in the Achilles tendon area, up to the middle of the calf of the leg. The patient lies face-down for this correction.

The tendon Achilles is the negative pole to the 4th lumbar and upward. The release of these energy blocks is essential in Sciatica, to free the sciatic nerve impulses.

EVOLUTIONARY SERIES

Stone also felt that work on the Achilles tendon area had a direct effect on the cortex and brain function.

In the chart opposite he also refers to the importance of the Achilles area and the base of the skull as being two weak areas in the body that need to be released frequently.

CHART
NO. 12

SUPERIOR-INFERIOR VITAL
BALANCING

FIG. 1 illustrates a contact with the right hand in a firm grip on the heel bone, with the thumb above and the index finger below. The left hand is on the occiput and atlas area. Top and bottom are being balanced. Both are weak spots & need release often.

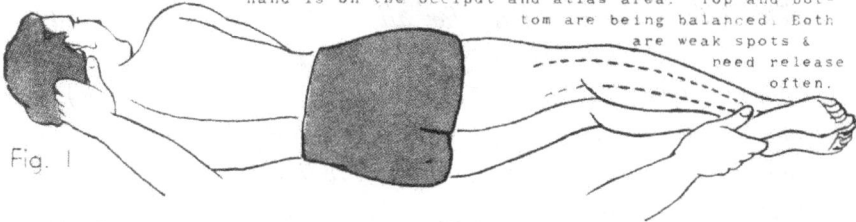

Fig. 1

FIG. 2 shows how any area on the calf of the leg, the leg, or the heel can be treated and balanced from a side position, while the doctor sits down. The thumb contact is firm in both applications. Sacral and Occipital contacts can also be made in this position.

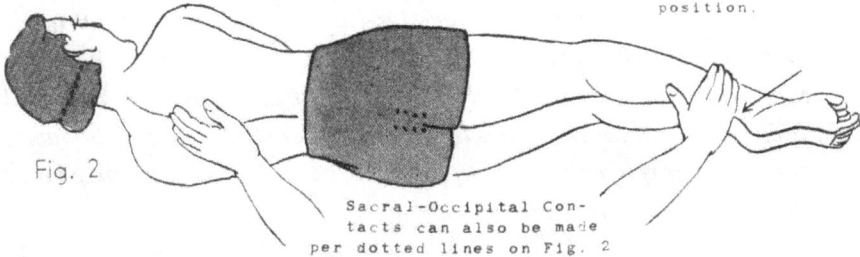

Fig. 2

Sacral-Occipital Contacts can also be made per dotted lines on Fig. 2

In the seminars Stone gave in the 1970s he often explained or elaborated on the charts in his books. When discussing charts 14-16 in his book 'The Wireless Anatomy of Man' which are reproduced from Varma's book 'The Human Machine and its Forces,' he spoke of a meeting he had with the British naturopath Stanley Lief, whom we have already met in relation to the creation of European NMT, and a discussion around Varma's work ensued. The meeting he refers to in the transcription below probably took place in the late 1950s or early 1960's. The bracketed additions in the two sets of quotes below are not in the original recording and are simply added for clarity.

"I showed this picture (showing a chart from Varma's book reproduced in Stone's 'Wireless Anatomy of Man') to Dr Lief, he was here from

England he is a naturopath at the big sanatorium there, he is known all over England. He is an authority on nature cure. I showed him this picture and I said it (the Varma book) was out of print, I did not know the man but I knew he was an Indian and that it was out of print, he (Dr lief) said yes I paid for all of that, he (Varma) did the experimenting and I (Dr Lief) paid the bills and he said he was glad I had it (the book) because it was absolutely useless he (Dr Lief) could not use it and he was not going to continue with it, it was pretty hard to peddle it, you see what they did was to find the sore spots here and then he worked on them, this man, this Indian, he actually worked out the sore spot but it was so darned painful nobody could take it. It was like working with direct leverage instead of working on the eliminative principle of the currents, and he (Dr Lief) said they could not use it (the Varma technique), but they could see these dark lines how this material becomes absolutely stagnant and becomes a material resistance. And the normal is this, that's the muscular tissue. (Showing the pranograph charts from Varma's book reproduced in Stone's 'Wireless Anatomy of Man')"

Stone – Seminar August 1973 [2]

Stone made some small additions to the charts he reproduced from Varma's book, the most notable being on the chart opposite where he adds some anatomical cell structure diagrams and other comments.

Referring to some of these additions Stone said:

"Here is a muscle cell and here is a connective tissue cell, each one has a different arrangement, the muscles cell has its centre here and expands this way and the connective tissue cell has a certain amount of elasticity in each fibre but it is not expansive like the muscles cell and that is the conductor, the connector from the power to the piston - the expansion is the piston.

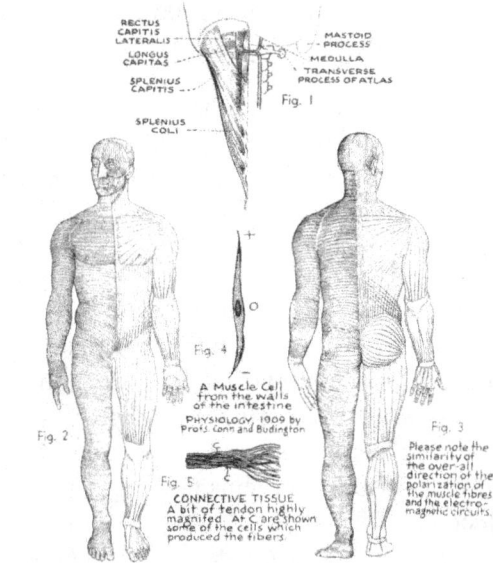

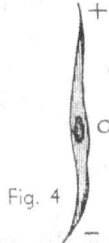

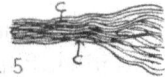

Now there was an apparatus made (showing a picture of the pranograph to students) by which you could picture the shades among the waste products in the system, wherever they saw this there is the way the muscle and the tissue have this waste product in it and it shows in the picture (showing pranograph pictures)"

Stone - Seminar August 1973

A study of Varma's book 'The Human Machine and its Forces' will show that the connective tissue per se was not something he was concerned with, his focus being on nerve and muscle. Though having said that in his other writings it is clear that he also took a broader view of treatment, he wrote:

"Very often it is a nerve, or rather a nerve cell (nervicule) welded to the muscle and, because of the unnecessary muscle

57

tissue there, it stopped transmitting its vibrations and therefore heat and movement. At other times, it is an organ that has moved slightly, oh! so slightly that we have every excuse for not being aware of it!

Here is a common case: 'the displacement of the aorta, the unknown cause of a host of diseases.' He who has studied only on cadavers cannot be as fully aware as one who has studied on his own body the exact and immutable position that it must occupy in the body.

But the past master in our method must be able to identify immediately, with no other instrument than his fingers, the slight shift and the necessary result, to correct the position of the organ. A simple, though infinitely delicate operation, which to a casual observer looks like a massage, but in the end, will remove very serious problems the origin of which was lost in conjecture.

Let us, in conclusion, give a kind of schema of our treatment. Here is the main outline, without further comments:

1. Nervous vitality must be restored throughout the body.

2. To do this it is essential to:

a) Put all of the organs in their place.

b) Return the nerves and the nerve fibers to their normal flexibility.

c) Re-align and relax the complete skeleton but mainly the vertebral column.

3. We must identify the location of the illness by palpation, assisted sometimes by auscultation (listening with a stethoscope) and percussion (the latter operation is accomplished without the aid of any instrument).

4. The revitalization of nerves and nerve centers by the dynamic action and vibration from the hands of the operator and his hands only.

5. General relaxation massage intended primarily to activate the circulation, this is an additional operation of real usefulness, but having only the value of an accessory factor in the work of healing.

The human body is a machine which anyone who claims to cure must be able to put all the pieces back as a watchmaker does a watch.

As long as a limb, or an organ is not removed from the body, the hope of a cure is still intact. The Reconstructive power of life is unlimited. It is sufficient to know how to put it in motion."
— The Key to Health Dewanchand Varma[3]

The connective tissue and the related energies are, as noted earlier, important in connection to our internal sense of self but also to something greater, something beyond the self. This was recognised by another pioneer in manual therapy Dr Andrea Rabagliati. In the opening quote at the beginning of this chapter Rabagliati refers to the link between the connective tissue and the ether. This linkage is a perception that Stone would have heartily endorsed.

In his book Initis[4] Rabagliati also wrote

"To say that the connective tissues connect every part of the body with every other is to give them a high place in function, since this is only another way of saying that they are the structures used by the force of life to act as the means by which the feeling of unity and solidarity shall be experienced in the animal body. ....

It is by the functional action of the connective tissues that we know without being told, and without requiring to be told, that every part of the body , however unimportant it may seem, belongs to the body and forms part and parcel of it.

Within our felt sense of the connective tissue is the dance of inner and outer, our sense of internal unity as well as our oceanic sense of connection with everything that exists outside of the self.

Finally, it is worth noting that the transcripts of the seminar lectures that I have included in this chapter come from the same time period covered by the Stone notebooks that follow. This should allow you to be able to trace the evolution of some of his later ideas on energy, consciousness and the connective tissue.

DR RANDOLPH STONE

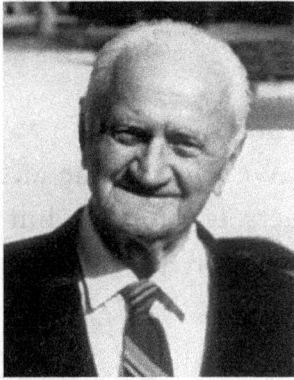

NOTEBOOKS
1970 -1973

FIRST NOTEBOOK

Dera, Jan. 1970.

Minnie's Reception; a Marvellous display of Arrangements of Lights - cleanliness in all the Dera = scrubbed. Marvellous planning and attention to every detail by Maharaji. About 40 invited Guests, accommodated all over the Dera for the night of the 6th, and the 7th all day. Weather was cold last night. The tents were decorated beautifully even. Charcoal heaters placed between tables.

There was some delay because the train was late. But everything went off beautifully. We came home after 10 pm., when the Guests had their dinners. It was cold - but lovingly told. About 1,000 persons were there in all - and hundreds could not be seated but stood all around.

It was a strenuous day for Maharaji. He had only 1½ hours sleep the night before.

Dera, Jan 6th, 1970. 2.30 am

1. The Hourglass of Energy flow.
2. The Zodiac Clock Dial ✝ Weather Vane.
3. Pressure on Zones ✛ Elemental Energy.
4. Time indicator, hour-hand - the Tamas substance, Tattwas – Jin (*Editor?*) form-Mind.

The Minute hand, the Pranas the Impulse changes - sensation and ideas indicated on the face of the Dial on all the body, facial expression walk, talk, action and responses.

Pressure on nerve ending circuits is like stepping on your Toes; it gets attention = the Attention Current, where the Consciousness is and acts. The child's cry knows this instinctively - and it gets attention.

Consciousness is at play all day as time stalks in play.

Dera, Jan 8th 9.30 pm 1970.

The Well of Humility:
1) Humility is like a Well,
In its empty space it can dwell.
The deeper it is, the more it can hold
Of the Lord's Grace, for humility to unfold.

2) As the full ear of grain bends low,
It really is humilities bow,
Which by the Creators design
Worships at the deepest shrine.

3) Its useful grain is its shield,
There are no glances to Vanity to yield.
Service and loyal devotion
Are its integrated life Motion.

4) Humility is the fullness of the seeming void
Which the force in Creation has destroyed.
Humility conceals the Father's hidden Love
In His Eternal Wonder Region from above.

Dera, Jan 9th 1970.

A beautiful day. Maharaji just left for Sirsa, with Mother and Shoti in the Chevrolet, loaded full. The Wedding is over and Maharaji needs a change and some rest. The Dera was scrubbed and cleaned from bottom to top, even the trees were washed. The impossible was accomplished. The old shacks and vendors stalls were all torn down and a wide clean road fills its place, plus a new modern building in the shade of trees for serving hot drinks and snacks which they had before in those stalls. So everyone is happy and provided for with comfort and in clean surroundings.

It is like a miracle of Love for every one.

Love travels in graceful curves of beauty and artful expression of warmth & feeling everywhere in hearts and in Nature.

Whereas intellect and force are cold and travel in straight lines directly to the objective.

Dera, Jan 9th 1970 7 pm.

Class Polarity Treatment sitting up A p5.

The best Polarity Treatment for Digestion is given sitting up, with one hand working on that side of the Erector Spinal Muscles over the Laminae of the Vertebrae and the other hand supporting the Upper Chest and ribs plus the Shoulder joint, pushing it posterior. This is the true Opposite Polarity position not that side = Anterior = Posterior. Not from one side to the other.

It also helps belching feely and gas movements out of the tissues.

With this combination the doctor can work on the most

affected side of the digestion, all up & down the spine and shoulder blade - and go in deep with the soft cushion of the thumb repeatedly, digging out air locks in the lesions and over the ribs without adjustments. It allows more work to be done and more specifically effective. ,Even in injuries and it helps the breathing and relieves pain.

Dera, Jan. 20th 1970.

1. A simple New Approach to treatment sitting up - and also lying down by the simple pressure release under the base of the occiput near the center for the Sympathetic tension and pains along the spine and tendons, attached to the occiput.

The flexion leverage applied from the forehead contact at the bridge of the nose and held in flexion with fingers and thumb pressure right under the occiput near the center, upward on the sorest and tensest tendon and area. Change sides to reverse the Polarity contact of the hands and thumb.

2. The same procedure is done with a contact on the Temporal bones on each side, along the occiput - behind the ears. This is partly Parasympathetic as it takes in lateral lines (zones) away from the Central Spinal Area Control.

The table treatment is the same with a hold under the occiput for the Sympathetic Control by more contact flexion hold, on one side and a sensory control light hold, behind the jaw and ear on the 10th Cranial Nerve on the other side. It becomes a balancing effect on the Sympathetic and Parasympathetic action.

I was able to show some of this to Mahesh and he is giving the cook treatment for his right shoulder arthritis and pain, with a trembling hand. It is most interesting and helpful all around. He gives the cook and others the exercise treatment of flexion and extension in the doorway on the sills as well as the correct squatting postures. It helps them all, as I can't talk their language and they love it. Even the treatment with the Magnets.

This all seems like a new start, which keeps patients fit, and enables me to instruct others to do it, as well as their own stretchings.

3. I marvel at "His Grace"

And little Louise sets the pace, with her problems of pain and keen intuition. Her left shoulder and arm pains were a real puzzle; and no routine treatment would take hold anymore; even the lift was undesirable and wouldn't work. It took a deeper concept bold and simple - more specific, easier and more effective to help out now. Even the chronic sore feet, toes and calves and shin bone area of the colon is gradually letting go, without any change in diet.

All His Grace and self revealing itself in its intricate tension fields, areas, switches and holds to release it all.

By utilizing the Overall Wireless Concept more through the extremities, it has broadened the field of Therapy and made it more effective and complete, as well as more practical and useful.

4. As well as the New Yoga Principles of mere flexion and extension, holds in the Postures and simple moves, is a wonderful help to those who will use them, even for 5 minutes every day with thoughtful leisure relaxation. Two minutes for any one posture is enough. It does wonders and gives instant result and tension release. It will keep anyone fit that understands it and will do it.

This all is for the Public well being. The treatments are for doctors to give to patients to inspire them, to self help through application and less rich food. More natural, raw live food is the answer.

P.S. It is cool rainy weather and there is no electricity or light. But "His" helpful inspiration needs none of this external force. It supersedes it all.

I have less patients now, and time to think and train one or two others.

5. Mahesh loves it and it helps him to keep fit, and all the other servants from the Guest House, including the cook. He needed it badly.

Mahesh takes to this type of yoga postures like a duck to water and can even show my patients how they should be done. This is very helpful to me especially with the natives who can't talk English. The Hakim and servants included. I am grateful what it is doing for Louise. She needed help and I did not have the answer, so she just got make-shift treatments, when she found time to take them. That was no good and not enough. This all is like a revelation when it is given direct and by necessity, without any other things like electricity, etc.

I am seeing internal Miracles done by "His Grace" - which were needed by all who get them. Some foreigners included from Holland, England and America. It is no work to serve Him it is rather a revelation in the Mystery of Life applied daily.

Dera, Jan 21st 1970.

Pain control through the Sympathetic, from high up in the center of the head - the Sphenobasilar tension. Firm pressure with leverage and Polarity is the key. Leverage from the forehead or the opposite side, also the Parasympathetic 10th Cranial nerve.

Sitting up, it is the heel of the hand over the shoulder area of the 10th Cranial nerve that works well. It is more forceful sitting up, for belching also. Lying on the Table is more for lateral contacts and the Polarity current with less pressure. Both are excellent!

It is Art - not force.

When the Center is cleared, then the condition is resolved from Center to the Extremities of the fingers and toes = Acute & Chronic.

Dera Jan 21st 1970.

Quotes from the Bhagavata Purana.

Krishna and the Gopis

p.423. The Wise Man having not Egoism. They have nothing to gain by good or bad deeds. The Lord dwells in all Beings, and He is the Manifester of all the Senses.

p.441. Krishna is in the heart of all Beings as fire is in the heart of all Wood. He has no father, no wife - no sons no-one near or distant, no body - no birth no Karma.

Thought void of all Gunas, He seeks them for pleasure for the purpose of Creation.

Uddhavas message to the Gopis "You are not separated from me I am all pervading."

As the 5 elements enter into the composition of all beings, so I underlie Manas, Prana, the Bhutas and Indbyas and Gunas.

Dera, Jan. 21st.

Quotes from the Bhagavata Purana, cont.

p.441 "Sleeplessly therefore control the Mind. This is the final Reach of Yoga, and of Samkhya of Relinquishment, of Tapas, of Control of the Senses and of truth itself."

"The Mind dwells on the distant lover most."

p.443. There are 7 Sakamaya Puris, or places on top of Meru as well as 7 Miskamaya Puris. Sakamaya are regions where desires fructify, 7 Miskamaya or Moksha producing Puris.

p.475. Purusa is One. Jiva Prakritis or Para Prakriti are many. To Purusa Jiva must always be negative, however positive it may be to the forms of Apana - Prakriti. Purush is always Male. And to him Jiva Prakriti is always female.

p.445. The Umbrella is Brahmaloka. The 2 feet are above and below.

Kaanstubha light overpowers all other light. Namely - Surya, Agni, - Vak and Candra.

The four hands are Sattva, Rajas, Tamas and Ahamkara.

Sankha consisting of 5 Bhutas is held by the hand representing Rajas.

Cakra consisting of Manas is held by the hand representing Sattva.

Padma is the Universe, the Primal Maya, held by the hand of Tamas.

Gada is primal Vidya or wisdom held by the hand representing Ahamkara.

p 447. Krishna is the Antaryamin or inner Ruler of Beings.

Balrama is Sutratman, the Ego.

p.449. The Gopas are Devas.

Nanda is Supreme Bliss.

Yasoda is Mukti.

Maya is threefold - Sattvika is Rudra, Rajas is Brahma and Tamasa is

Daityas.

Devaki is Deva - ki chanted by them

Brahma vidya

Brahma is the stick of Krishna

Rudra is His flute.

Indra is His horn.

Gokula Vana is Vaikuritha

The Daity as (Tranvarta and others) are greed, anger, and other vices.

The trees are Rishis of Vaikuhtha.

Krishna in the form of Gopa is Hari.

Krishna is Paramatman in his relation to the Gopis.

p.450. The 8 principal queens and the 16,100 wives of Krishna are

Riksis and the Upanishads.

Canra is Duesa - (Dislike)

Mustika is Matsara (Egoism, Envy).

Kuvalayapida is Darpa (Arrogance)

Baka is Garva, (Pride)

Rohini is Daya, (Tenderness).

Satyabhana is Ahimsa (Non-injury).

Kamsa is Kali

Sudaman is Sama (Restraint of the Mind)

Akrura is Satya, (Truth)

Uddhava is Dama (restraint of the senses)

Sankha is Vishnu himself in the form of Lakshmi.

The milk products of the Gopis corresponds to the Ocean of Milk in the Universe.

The rope used in tying of Krishna is Adity.

Cakra is Veda

The Garland Vaijayanti is Dharma

The Umbrella is Akasha

Gada is the Goddess Kalika.

p. 451. The Lotus is the seed of the Universe. Garuda is the religious fig tree Bhandira.

A Gopi is she who preserves people from Naraka - from fear - & death. The Padma Purana throws the greatest light on the Brindavana Lila of Shri Krishna. The chapter refers to the Patala Khanda of that Purana.

Of innumerable Brahmandas (Solar Systems) there is one Supreme seat that of Vishnu. Of this seat Gokula is the highest aspect, and Davaraka Goloka

Varkuntha is , Swaloka and others the lower aspect.

71

There are several sub forests too, which witnessed scenes of other Krishna Lila.

The bow of horn (Sarnga) is the Maya of Vishnu.

The arrow is Kala, the destroyer of all lives.

The husk stand is the discrimination product faculty = husks from grains separated.

When all fruits are offered to Krishna there is a rich return. By surrendering the Ego, spirituality is now possible. "Deny yourself," said Jesus.

Dera, Jan. 22nd 1970.

Quotes from the Bhagavata Purana, cont.

p.502. Mula Prakriti in the universe, of Buddhi in Man, is wedded to Atman represented by Krishna.

p.465. Once more let us understand the triad - Adhyatma - Adhybhuta - and Adhideva. Take sight. The sense of sight comes in contact with the outside world and carries the perception of sight to the possessor of the eye, under the guidance of Conscious Energy.

The senses and the Mind are cows of Adhyatma. The outside world is grass of Adhubhta.

The possessor of the senses and the Mind is the Gopis, the Ego or Jiva. In Brindavan the Gopis are the highest Jivas of Rishis as expressed in the Upanishads.

p.465, cont. The conscious Energy is the Gopa or Adhideva; they are the Vedic Devas; the Gopas are reincarnation of the Devas. Ordinarily the Gopas lead the cows or the Adhidevas lead the senses; but in Brindavan the Devas surrender themselves entirely to Krishna.

p.466 The Calves, or the Vatsas are the modifications of the senses and the Mind - the Vrittis. The Lord tended the Vrittis of the Mind, therefore they could go astray.

[Vatsa (-asura) A demon friend of Kamsa's who entered Vraja in the form of a calf and was killed by Krishna.]

Baka the Crane stands for spiritual hypocrisy, spiritual life rejects all hypocrisy and untruth in any form.

Agha is sin - an evil deed. In their struggle the whole nature is changed - in a daily dying.

Dera - Jan. 22nd 1970 Definition of terms.

Gunas -

Inbuyas -

Bhutas -

Tanmatras -

Jantra -

Pencil notes on top of
THE HONG KONG HILTON
Asia's east meets west hotel -
notepaper.

April 17th 1972 Mill Valley.

The 3 guna actions and Karma [O] [+] [-]

The 3 nervous systems

The 3 types of treatment.

The cerebrospinal = <u>structure</u> - support and motion pains [-] negative - <u>air</u> and <u>earth.</u>

[+] positive = The sympathetic is the saman fire rajas – [+] <u>radiation, dilation fever,</u> heat - swelling, <u>muscular pain</u>, hallucius longus treatment, emotional release lock.

Water

[O] The parasympathetic is the neuter pole [O] - intestinal linings - diverticulitis, enteritis colitis - bad tongue & digestive needs neck rotation - perineal. Treatment - top – <u>10th Cranial & 11th</u> and heels outside & the hip over femur. Karmic pralab treatment (*"During our sojourn on the earth-plane, we work out our destiny or fate as planned with great precision and exactitude by what is called Pralabdh Karmas, which determine in broad outline the general framework marking the duration and course of life in each case. " by sant Kirpal Singh Ji. Editor*)., sterno clydo mastoid treatment.

The nervous patient - tense - gas - and fear.

74

2nd Day.

Rollers, balls, Libbies 5½ oz. cans filled with ice cubes or crushed ice - tied to ankles & under arches - on spine for low blood pressure - on thumb blood pressure treatment & squat. Dilators etc = through orifices.

Sitting up treatment - Head treatment = drain top

x neck - spine, gas angina & heart treatment

Yawns - belches etc. Gas release. The Sacred Flame. Sex is but the frame.

3 Vital Elements = Jewel -

4 Acupuncture & this needles - treatment principle

Body outlets = space energy

Body tendons = structure energy

Magnetic fields = parallel flow

3 gunas =   fire through the eyes –

Palms of hands -

Arches of feet -

Clean hands and pure heart. 3rd eye concentration.

Boraxo - then remedies rub in with thumbs in palms and over the back also with Boroxo (*Borax transposed over the word. Editor*).

Structure is the 5 elements of matter.

Function is the vital current of the energy of Sahansdal Kanwal as nature's element of Spirit and the soul power of awareness and Inner Realisation of spirit animation.

3rd Day. (*page torn. Editor*)

Red blood = Prana

Use postures for-the tattwa flow, moving gases - and fluid via Prana.

Neuter posture of embryo.

Use breath for prana flow - thumb pressure abdomen in & out - Udana and curved tongue inhale drop head - hold & out - for blood purification & high blood pressure. Bowel triangle (? *Editor*) drink air in and out. Respiration with abdominal movements.

Acu - puncture = current withdrawal = no sensation.

Light treatment. color = gases plasma.

5 elements in action revolving like a wheel = the swastika

Left hand unwinding   Right hand

whirl = negative [-]   Whirl = [+] Fiery tale

The cross in motion

flying disks - 4 tattwas center plus

the bulb of matter is the plasma

Gas - or the 5 subtle elements . Plasma

Sun = Radiation or spinning out hot gases and lava.

   +

Lib + Lib: Woman's space

= Iblis

Elaborate the 5 fingers and elements =

1st day - 3 gunas - 5 elements & prana - jeln (?) treatment.

magnets as energy force in treating the spine

2nd day Ball rollers - iced tomato cans + pressure, ice on ankles, ice under the arch

2,500 pores per sq. in. subtle gas escape thru 400 pores - for air exchange in skin-

2 currents from hands - arch and eyes. Heat to the arches and hands for pores opening.

1. Search 1. River = 4

   Energy used as a short cut to health.

2. Poems establish the principles of polarity.

   Energy must circulate

   The 3 gunas [O] [+] [-] 3 qualities

          V Br S

3. The 5 spiritual sounds

   5 pranas and 5 elements

   5 senses - motor & sensory.

   The 3 nervous systems.

   Circulatory - sympathetic blood O

   Cerebrospinal = lymph

   Parasympathetic = cerebrospinal fluid

   secreted in the ventricles of the brain

Magnets - push & pull energy by the choroid plexuses.

4. The Secret = energy circuits & plasma gas.

tendons & ligaments - hollow fibres = collagen fibres. Conductors of prana and plasma gas for movement of the structure

Vital force = prana moves all things in nature [-] [+]

gases [-] = chakras & tattwas

elements - have color and sound.

Show book & 5 circuits-

Treatment: show feet negative pole of psychic energy - soles of feet and hands

Gases flow out through the 2500 pores per square in on the palms of the hands and the 400 pores per square inch on the rest of the body.

Face down with pillow

Primary respiration

NOTES FROM DR STONE'S NATIONAL NOTE BOOK

NAME: Dr. Randolph Stone

SCHOOL: Life

CLASS: A

Polarity Therapy is different from Acupuncture and Shiatsu. Why – O

on the back name and publisher etc of Health and Vitality at Your Fingertips.

Dera Jan 1973

Life's Golf Game

Life's Game of Golf

1.Hit the Ball and let it roll
2.Hit it hard right at the Goal
3.Follow it with a leisure stroll
And finish putting at the holes.

Life's Objectives are the Ball
Once hit, they are beyond recall.

His Will & Destiny.

1)Only Thou canst decree
What each particle shall be.
Only thou dost know
Where each one shall go.

2)The yearning of each Soul
Lies engraved in thy Scroll
To fulfil each part in its heart
The whole Creation did Start.   .

3)To express the Whole,
Each needed a Soul
as God's messenger
and Creation's goal.

4)The Essence of Bliss
Know itself as His
and now its radiance trapped
in to precious stones enwrapped

5)The rays still and fine
But the Soul doeth pine
And cry as for lost
"Thou and Thine," me and mine.

6)The need and creed
Are hollow indeed
And the Life Breath wails
Thru its selfless entrails

7)Being nought of the ought
In Love and in Thought
On Being and seeing
The Soul Itself freeing

8) Light and Love was wrought
as a Mighty drought
and poured into Creatures
Giving them form and features

9) In this, Life's sacred Stream
Lies the Song and its Theme
The hidden Glory of His in all in that is,
Unknown, unsung and unseen.

Nirat is most important to practice - 1st Light - then Sound. It precedes. As long as the bulb is not screwed into the socket, the electric can give no light.

Dera Jan. 17th 1973.

1st sunshine.

Outline of the Principles of Polarity.

Creation ... Immensity of overflowing Love - from the *Atman* state of Bliss Concentred Essence.

The Story of the Soul = the royal rays - spark and jewel of all creation. Wrapped up in various states densities as crystallizing energy and light essence from the world - the Shabd Sound Current eternally concealed in the bosom of the Father unrevealed.

The 3 gunas as qualities △ ♈ ○ + —

The 5 elements as tattwas - subtle and gross - unseen matter essence - sensory and motor energy.

2. The 5 tattwas = the play of matter as substance and light radiation of colours - and friction sound of matter plus the unseen sense play by which the natural creation note - attracts and repels - - - It calls and communicates between creatures in the wild - attracts them for propagation - without any outer organization or communication governed by the Sun & Moon - time element and climate - not by will - or choice of their own.

Subtle sense development keener than man's - guide and protect the unconscious play of life - and nourishment by attraction & repulsion.

The [-] space action and [+] matter substance occupying space.

3. The pranas as the unconscious energy of the Sun and Moon play – arising and ascending in the sap of all vegetation with Sun currents and return*ing* to the earth ⌒↘ after its zenith - noon time - attracted by the earth's position of repose.

See the atom's etheric whirls in ◯ Babbits 1971 notes. Also tattwas in color. The aura - radiation of matter and substance. It is all in the notes and in my books in detail but it must be a living unit - a whole that is integrated - felt and understood so it becomes a self directed realization - with a clear view for Therapy application of O + -.

4. The Mind:

Guru Sawan Singh said : The Mind is the Sattva guna essence of the 5 tattwas, activated by the current of the Spirit. It is superior to the tattwas, but inferior to the conscious current. It represents the intermediate state. — (between the tattwas and the soul). Get rid of the 3 covers: material, astral, causal and thus rises above the 3 gunas (qualities) and the 5 tattwas, then the 25 prakritis, mind and maya and reaches Par Brahm, then he realises that he is a pure Soul = to the effulgence of 12 suns.

5. Acting from the center out is natural expression for each chakra subtle and gross space of the 5 elements or central centers of the tattwas.

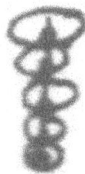

Cause is energy and consciousness expressing itself in effect.

Action must flow harmoniously - not be mere exercise.

In Radha Soami Science, the Gurus uses the Shabd - the Soul energy and Mind to unfold the Inner Consciousness.

Not prana: as this is unconscious energy in nature's unfolding process following the sun energy rays up and currents of the moon ⫯ down day and night - crown and root system.

Dera. Jan. 18th 1973.

For Blood Pressure and Sugar

Neck treatment of sympathetic & parasympathetic. The lesion in the spinal articulation over the lamina and the 10th cranial parasympathetic nerves on each side anterior along the sternocleidomastoid muscle. Tension release here is via the lightest touch - - - in back of neck, the sympathetic is pressure support - - - hold both to balance.

In the tension chemicals of high blood pressure - or sugar and in asthma and respiratory problems all this is vital and delicate – effective: Naidu & Dhingra

Dera, Jan. 20th 1973.

Explanation is for the Mind: Inspiration and vision is for the Soul. "My people perish for lack of vision" said Lord Jehovah to Moses on Mount Sinai. The Tisra Til vision center; [*3rd eye*] the mark on the forehead - in the Bible - from Genesis. Chap 4 v 15 to Revelations.

Nod East of Eden. v.16 Cain's son was Enoch - 7 fold- revenge.

Dera Jan. 30th 1973.

W*orking the* toe tips *is* a special treatment for parasympathetic treatment of subtle conditions of nerve tension symptoms from the head. Like burning sensation in the bottom of the feet or water sensation for Naidu. Treating through socks or bare toe pulling with the special latex holder. 3 points on the toe, the tip is for the brain cortex tension. And the tips and nails are sensitive to pressure. It is a special approach for difficult cases that are hard to find the answer to *as well as for* subtle complaints.

Dera Jan. 30th 1973.

Pleurisy Naidu. Special work on the upper dorsals with shoulder leverage and effort - lying on the side, also sitting up.

Gave Louise a complete sitting up treatment... treatment for head drainage - shoulders, back and springing the spine.

Dera Feb. 1st 1973.

To move gases and gas pressure in the circulation and the bowels use oil in hot soup, or broth, plain olive or sesame oil - about 6 tablespoonfuls in 3 cups of hot soup - nothing else - repeat.

Feb. 1st 1973.

Manjh was a very wealthy man, who became a disciple of Guru Amar Das [*actually his son Guru Arjan Dev Ji. Editor*] - who put him to the severest tests possible - and he went thru it faithfully (with his wife.)

Then, as a favor he asked that no other disciple be put thru such ordeals before acceptance to Initiation. We all owe him a big thank you!

Dera Feb. 6th 1973 8.30 am.

Not so cold a nice day: Maharaji left about 7am in a rush. He wanted no-one to see Him off. He said he would call before leaving. Naidu and Louise went there to get His Darshan and help with loading the car, and Louise wanted to be there if there was a forgotten message of some dictation. She got it.

Feb. 6th 1973 8.30 am.

1 Khajuraho and 2 Konarak; a comparative study. 1 in Madhya Pradesh

2 in Orissa.

Feb. 12th 1973.

Dera - warmer weather.

A series of sitting up treatments with table treatment.

Head treatment. Occiput & Sphenobasilar treatment, Spinal spring - etc.

The Deluxe Polarity Squat - 10 min - 3 times a day - to break the prana tension fields and release the plasma gas pockets. ○ through the pores.

Specific in diet to help this along is mehti as greens - and or cooked with onions and mehti dona (fenugreek) seeds in herb tea.

March 3rd 1973 - Dera.

Sin unexpressed, is a sin obsessed,
Sin exposed is a sin dispossessed.

From Indian Spiritual Pictorial Diary 1973.

March 6th 1973 Dera.

1973 Readers Digest quote from Robert Houdini's tricks in "Maestro in the Magic Circle". In Algeria he exposed every trick in the marabouts' arsenal. He shows that how by rubbing their tongue and soles with Alum and soap they are able to swallow live coals and walk on red hot iron bars.

Dera March 7th 1973 6am.

A spheno-basilar adjustment through the side of the bridge of the nose with the head tilted in the squatting position.

New - two definite clicks in the head. Personal experience.

Dera March 9th.

Camile is leaving today. The Texas chiropractor - broken coccyx = spheno-basilar opposite [+] pole relieved. She is a real buster.

The osteopath from South Africa and his problem of excess perspiration cause unknown. It was indigestion found under the left floating ribs

Tongue shows intestine and transverse colon inflamed. He was well pleased *and* wants to come to America for my class there.

Dera, March 10th 1973.

A new Ying & Yang treatment.

Indigestion creates gas pressure in the temples *with* throbbing *swollen* veins.

From DR STONE'S GREEN NOTEBOOK.

Nov. 24th, 1972 - Dera.

Brief Notes on Polarity:

The River of Life flows as fine Etheric Energy over the organs of speech - senses and internal functions.

Shabd and Surat are Current like, and flow from their Center or Source fulcrum support.

The Anterior of the body is sensory and receptive.

The back of the body is Motor and repelling.   Mercury ☿

The Center stream is a Neuter Current - The Shushmana, or Tchi.

The Middle Vertical line - which yang and Yin divides into ♈ 2 branches

⧖ Superior   Anterior Positive. + & — Right & Left.
⧗ Inferior

1. The One River divides into 4 Tattwas *or* essences of ☮ Matter.

The 5 Pranas are the Life Energy blended with the 5 elements as Tattwas and flow thru them as Tchi or Life and all sense combinations as Vital Energy and Substance or essence, making the internal secretions in their chemical laboratory of glands - these enzymes are the genes of Life's pattern after that kind each

In the body:

Superior - the Crown

Middle - the Life secretion of sustenance

Bottom - the generation and roots of Mind = Matter.

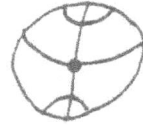

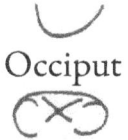

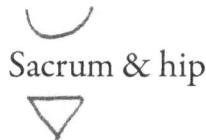

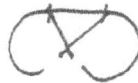

Occiput   Sacrum & hip

heels on sides and Centre line.

2. Sympathetic centers - along the Lamina Neck Sympathetic lesions. Parasympathetic *centers* are 10th and 11th Cranial. Anterior Sensory & Cerebrospinal Nervous system. Vertebral and 3 pairs of nerves. Sore spinous processes & hyperemia. Laminal lesions - tensions.

Spinal Treatment & Gas = Connective Tissue

White Circulation of lymph - cerebrospinal fluid through tendons & ligaments.

Muscular Circulation is = Red - Iron Core

Haematin or Haemoglobin = the Yang fluid

Connective tissue is white = Magnesium

Core or vegetable - or Vegetative Circulation

the Yin fluidic conductor of Prana

Vital sap fluid = White penetration where the red muscle tissue ends.

Cellular fire and water sap as life enzymes with vitamins.

Dera, Dec. 6th 5.AM. 1972.

Sheet on Levine and Magicore.

Spinal Treatment *focusing* on 4th lumbar for Gas.

Testing sensitive spinous processes.

Treat against greatest resistance - and less painful

Have patient face down over pillows to raise

the Lumbars, use the legs as levers - for flexion stress and extension foot leverage, with vertebral contacts instead of adjustment.

It is the vital force of Prana circulation as Tchi that must ! penetrate all tissue cells to give life and motion - flow*ing* in and out ! [+] & [-] Yang penetration out, Yin Relaxation *in*.

Sperm cell motion and ovum embrace .

Sitting up treatment on legs doubled under brings out the lower spine and *moves the* sacrum *posterior* ! gives more leverage and hold. A Special Treatment.

5.30 am.

The same Connective Tissue Principle Mystery – White & Red - Circulation carried into the spinal vertebrae and their ligaments as the real tension lesions and cause of subluxated vertebrae *needing* treatment.

- *circulation* carried thru red tissues as life function = expansion and contraction - white = Life ⭕ Current flow ⭕ or oval circuits in atoms and cells.

5 Elements = tattwas reflection of 5 spiritual regions

5 senses - both motor [+] and sensory [-]

3 gunas = space motions

3 nervous systems

3 densities = solids, salt - liquids, mercury and gaseous matter, sulphur.

2 pairs of opposites - fire [+] Water [-]

2 pairs of opposites supporting the subtle air and gross earth

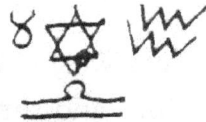

♓ Pisces 2 fishes = currents tied together by tail

Poor Richard Almanack published by Benjamin Franklin.

Look for fishes on shin bone in my book page 64 Wireless Anatomy of Man.

Vital Life Current of Generation - the Water Energy of Pisces.

Precipitation.

Sensory = Concentration - Coagulation.

Dera. Dec 7th 1972.

Wu-Wei - Easy Stretch for Heart and leg pains

Have arms shoulders 22" length

Stand in front of bed, with hands on bedstead - squat way down - relax - to lift the upper ribs and shoulders.

Then push away from the bed hold forward to stretch the leg tendons and the calves *to* get the gas out.

The feet bear all the weight and do not change positions at all.

There is no strain whatever in the posture or in the forward push and back for low relaxation.

The Udana exhalation lift can be added for upward air current exhalation and pelvis muscle *activation* to complete the inner lift.

Dec 7th 6.30 am.

This Wu Wei neuter position stretches the yang and the yin end positions and the Tchi in the center that is free rather than a fixed fulcrum or a lever only.

It includes the secret of all posture = effortless flexibility.

It stretches all tendons tenderly - without stretching - by merely shifting position .....

Wu Wei = body weight shift = no stress or effort, or support changes from the feet - only slight flexion and extension over the ankle leverage.

It is as subtle as holding the Mind still in its own effortless way, while moving the cables of Tchi = the Center's subtle life equilibrium. Neuter in Space near the Spirit Ace. The Atom of Motion.

Dec. 7th.

The Secret of the Perpetuation of the human Race - locked in Space - and ravished in its own place.

A Vacuum that draws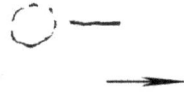

and an Arrow with Claws

The Consciousness of the Whole

Lies in the secret of the Soul.

Who can approach that Dragon tree?

Only the pure Soul, that itself is free.

Sex is but the frame

Of the Sacred flame.

The Rose of life in its color and lines of Grace-

That Maya of beauty attracts in every place.

Life's magnetic charm,

Love and arm,

Locked in

Dec. 8th. 1972 Dera.

Chetan = Spirit = mood

It is the spirit that enlivens and inspires "The flesh profiteth nothing". (*John 6:63*)

Interest with concentrated effort is the real Art of Genius and Inspiration by directing the concentrated attention current with natural skill in any undertaking or learning a profession. Life discovers itself in action as proof. The mood or the 3 fates guide the subtle threads of Life's expression. Music without inspiration is dead.

Service without love is work.

Ability and skill are developed by effort and experience, not by talk.

93

The subtle Energy Currents unseen are the five fine points of Causes that produce the effects in Wu Wei postures and in Polarity Therapy. Feeling energy flow. Effortless effort is Art.

Dera. Dec.12th 1972.

Ligamentous Stretch

1. Special Treatment for Sacrum release - for the primary Respiration rhythm of the brain as expansion and contraction.

2. For leg trouble, tendon spasms, heel pains, cramps in legs etc. (Bulakami 8.45 AM. treatment)

Treat 1st with the shoulder stretch - hanging from a table with arms supported 22"apart $\longmapsto$

Thumbs support.

Squat reach $\longrightarrow$ forward to stretch heel tendons and calves of legs - back - and sacrum, sit there for tendon stretch. Feel it - attention current is the secret in all Yoga. 493 - Vol II Sar B. [*unknown book reference*]

Exhale with Udana lift - open the path of the *Sound* Current from Sahansdal Kanwal [*the region of the thousand-petaled lotus*] to Sacrum.

All this is effortless effort - let it flow without strain or self action.

Muscle stretch with foot leverage from the box or step; a fall on - syp. [*unclear reference*]

Dera, Dec. 18th 1972.

Indriyas = senses

Gunas = qualities

Stretch the back also - via the abdominal holds & air

Abdominal Treatment ⇄ on the fat and external muscles.

↑ ↑ and under the diaphragm - roll it up - and squeeze the fat.

Vishnu or Hari (the Preserver)

Shiva or Hara (the destroyer)

The long trek to the holy *Sabari Hills* by devotees of the Lord

Ayyappa the deity presiding of the Sabari Hills in Karala.

The pilgrimage itself is symbolic of the soul's journey to unite with the Supreme, the Summum Bonnum of Life.

Dec. 21st 1972 Dera.

Louise's specific treatment. Short and effective.

Sitting up on the table. *A lift plus* 4th lumbar and Sacral release.

Sitting lower on a chair - for neck release and lift of occiput stretch.

Then bend forward with elbows or arms on knees - to get the spine to give like a stretch to each area - and without adjustment all up and down the spine.

Dec. 22nd 1972.

Shila's specific treatment with a thumb contact on the center of the head - for Tchi circuit (felt in abdomen with fingers on side of head as a pull as in craniopathy!)

Hand on throat and one on top of head for "tension."

Dera, Dec 22nd 1972.

A copy from classical Greece, Time & Life Books; page 101 refers to Euripides in the Trojan woman, Adromache, the Trojan princess, relinquishes her small son to be killed by the Greeks with these words.

Thou little thing
That curlest in my arms, what sweet scents cling
All around thy neck! Beloved; can it be
All nothing, that this bosom cradled thee
And fostered; all the weary night where through
I watched upon thy sickness, 'til I grew
Wasted with watching? Kiss me. This one time.
Not ever again. Put up thine arms and climb
About my neck. Now, kiss me, lips to lips ....
O, ye have found an anguish that outstrips
All tortures of the East, ye gentle Greeks!

Dera, Jan 9th 1973.

A warm day with sunshine. -

Maharaji is in Sirsa; he left 7am Jan. 6th.

You wrote Pierre - that you would give ½ day time to explain the [+] and [-] sign positions in tracing currents - gross and subtle. Also explain the gross cavities - like chest and abdomen and the subtle energy currents of mind and emotional body which permeate them.

Vertical line up - meeting horizontal tattwa resistance.

Hands - inside and out - abdomen - calves - tissue type cross over - anterior and posterior soft and hard. [*A reference to the soft tissue on the abdomen relating to the soft tissue on the back of the thighs and calves -see Stone Polarity Therapy Vol II, Vitality Balance, Chart 3 page 32 and page 46, 6th paragraph. Editor*]

General overall currents & local aura radiation like electrons

2. Also ½ day of the neck treatment technique of draining the head – sitting up.

Local opposition in the technique for sore spots anterior & posterior and for *hot* & cold applications. Treating the spine sitting up.

A treatment for Colds. Garlic & Honey - & Lemon for hoarseness and sore throat, and lymph stasis anywhere.

Breast lumps *treated with* Perineal and buttocks contacts *gives good* response. Very light touch on anterior side - or affected side for circuit balance.

Meridians and Zones - as paths for life's energy travel in the sap - of trees.

[+] and[-] outside surface path - shell and bark

middle neuter - soft kernel

core - nutmeat

needles under the skin in sub dermal - as into the ascending tree sap under the bark.

Yin and Yang opposite sides and leverage with neuter fulcrum. Hollow organs and solid organs as a trace of energy - for acupuncture points.

Meridians differ from zones of the 5 senses and 5 tattwas radiations from 5 fingers and toes anterior & posterior

The Life Energy Currents and its distribution and cross over points.

The 5 elements of matter – the tattwas - the 4 humors ----

The 5 senses and their outlets in fingers and toes - and 5 oval sweeps overall currents anterior & posterior as zones or vertical meridians [-] [+]

Horizontal meridians ⟋ anterior posterior - side to side - right to left.

Diverting the current with a needle in its path - or to increase the current of vital force - overcoming gas blocks, *there are* 2 kinds *of gas* CO_2 & plasma

Dera Jan 9th 1973 6 pm.

Treatment to Louise, for a very sore spot in the occiput on the left. 1st head drain - strong lift - loosens gases later when you work the spine on both sides, up and down, patient sitting up straight on the table - a whip movement - rocking.

Or sitting on a chair bent forward with elbows on the knee giving a free spring to the spine.

Always try to find the lock of the intelligent current of attention - free it.

Lying on table - try north pole stretch. Then use local technique for the occiputal sore spot and atlas - by lifting up the neck with the finger tips and gentle stretch with tension.

The gas release relieves the soreness

Dera Jan 10th. 1973 12.15am.

Wrapped in kindness and amaze
In Sat Gurus loving grace.

Dera Jan. 10th 1973 3.30 pm.

<u>A unique ankle aid</u> and stretch on the heel - with a pull contact on the <u>top of the foot</u> - extending it downward. Thumb on fingers outside of heel pull.

Dera Jan. 12th 1973 3am.

<u>No Starches Cure.</u>

Poor Starch digestion *is* a gas problem that is not understood around the world, resulting in terrible headaches, abdominal gas pains, throbbing temple arteries and indigestion, all over *the body, it causes* gas pockets and pains *in the hips* — legs, etc.

The Cause *is* injury to the digestive system, by poison in water or food (mustard gas during the War for example) *even* strong medicine given to remove worms or poison *can do it, in fact,* anything that weakens the power of digestion. Then the starches eaten ferment daily and that is not understood anywhere even at Mayo's Clinic. Cases proved it.

Dera, Sat. Jan. 13th 1973.

Headache and gas in the head Treatment.

Use Pressure on each side of the head, sitting up - in a gentle lift, and fingers working slowly over top of the head - bring out the gas blocks beneath as belches and relief.

Yin [-] & Yang [+] Treatment under ribs.

Shushmana Canal of Sound Current from Sahansdal down to end of Sacrum.

Dera, Tues. Jan. 16th 1973.

Principles and aphorisms explained in the Radha Soami sacred writings.

1. What is Mind?

Master, Sawan Singh says (March 11. 1940 Discourses). Mind is the sattwa guna, essence of the five tattwas, activated by the current of the spirit. It is superior to the tattwas, but inferior to the conscious current. It represents the intermediate state between the tattwas and the Soul. The whole world worships Mind. We are all ruled by Mind in all our relationships and actions. Mind and Maya reaches to Par Brahm, Sunna region of Daswan dwar.

2. When you cross the til chakra, (blue curtain), you will see Jyoti. It has got 1,000 lights.

Master: the prana force has no consciousness. It is jar, lifeless pronounced (jwr).

The Mind and all thinking end and you listen to Akath - Katha - the tale that cannot be related. That is the endless Song.

1. *Veins standing* out on the temples with excess perspiration *and* wet hands and cold feet *is an* all Yang & Yin current flow block, that can be reached from under the floating ribs on each side. A brand new hold not just pressure or motion.

It is part of the Shah Rag or Shah Rug, literally the Royal Vein (*or life Chord*) *which is* the central current or canal in the finer body = it is called Shushmana or Sushumna which is the central current in the spinal column.

2. To the left is called the Ida - or Ira or Yin - and on the right side known as the Pingala or Yang. The key to indigestion and head trouble - gas and eyes and skin reflexes - eczema etc is wetness.

Dera - March 12th 1973.

A lovely day. The 3 Gunas are the Tchi - the Yin and Yang. The Astral body is the vital current from the head region, the △ Fontanel or the 1000 Petalled Lotus of light rays which animates it as well as all the Universe.

Vital Energy is the Key of Life and Health.

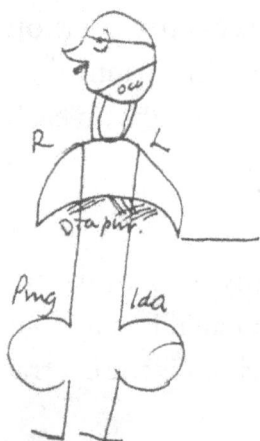

The Crown. The Pattern World of the ideas and Mind action, Parasympathetic Nervous system.

Air = Oxygen and Plasma heavy gases - electrically charged positive or negative

For negative *pole* block treat the Central Life current of Vital Energy from above - release it under the ribs near the center area - as a gas block.

2. The feet and the negative pole - the crystallized energy and sedimentation.

The Yin pole

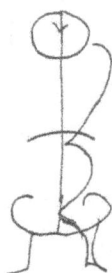

Superior = Shiva - Shrichtra (?)

treating the 3 gunas + mental

middle = vishnu   vital Yang Yin respiratory.

Inferior = Brahma - genitals. + breasts + feet

(two fishes tied together)

(two fishes tied together)

Dera. March 30th 1973.

Hot and cold shower 1st.

Lemon & hot tea - for sweating every half hour - 2 hours.

Perspiration in excess is Indigestion.

The 5 tattwas and pranas are natures gears to perform physiological functions thru tissues, via poles [O] [+] [-] and leverage flexion and extension.

Connective tissue holds the secret of the water relationship of respiration to structural motion via the tendons and ligaments – by the lymph and cerebrospinal fluid passing through the collagen fibres of the connective tissues.

The red lion of fire and circulation - stops at the tendon - or ligament, and the lamb - the white lymph takes over carrying with it the cerebrospinal fluid.

The energy of Prana must get through plasma gas blocks in tissue which are locked. CO_2 must be moved out of cellular lesions also, by manipulation.

Dera, April 3rd 1973.

A quote from the Weekly of India Magazine. Apr 1st.

"How magnetic storms are caused: The Sun is important to our planet, because solar radiation is responsible for plant and animal life, food, weather and climatic changes. Solar electromagnetic radiations also ionises the upper atmosphere of the earth, which makes long distance short wave communication possible.

When the sun is quiet, the wind travels outward from the sun and with a velocity of about 300-400 km per second.

2. A sudden release of plasma by solar flares causes a blast wave of solar particles which travel outward at 1,000 km per second. The collision of the solar wind with the magnetic field of the earth causes magnetic storms, auroral display and acceleration of particles in the Van Allen Radiation Belt."

April 10th 1am Dera – 1973.

Exercise *can activate* prana circulation. It starts from the root of the spring of the step - the elasticity of movement and leverage over the 5 tattwas of matter.

Sitting up and holding the toes, with sole contacts as fulcrum - let the ankle movement of the feet be the action and fulcrum factor. The resistance comes from the opposite poles of hands- arms- shoulders & back - to distribute the prana over the plasma gas blocks of emotions and mind pattern resistance which is the plasma gas radiation block from opposites.

2. The primal protons and electrons and carry great heat - 630 million units of fahrenheit for nuclear fusion and fission in the creative process. And in miniature in our own emotions and mind actions.

The Prana is the essential, physical vital force which is the virtue of plants and all vegetation and things and animals. It is the circulating finer, (the ever becoming) Energy thru the 5 tattwas or elements. Prana is the unconscious force in all creation and in nature. It links with the air and heavy gases like plasma for materialization of energy into bodies and forms.

3. Prana is the force that sprouts in the seed - or slumbers in its shell for ages - until acted upon by nature – *the* Sun's warmth and the moon's coolness in its time and season, in an earthy form or body. The mechanics are the same in a seed of a weed, or grain - or a mosquito or an elephant. All moved by prana in time and space. Prana is the real nourishment in food besides the matter bulk of minerals and water and air.

4. Stretching the connective tissues from the toes up 5 fulcrum levers through the ankle movement of push and pull - the flexors and extensors or tendons do the trick and establish the circuit of energy flow - the real object of stretching.

Choroid plexuses secret.

The secret lies in the tendon as the lymph and cerebro-spinal fluid circulation via the collagen fibres in the tendons or ligaments which link the bones and muscular action in a unit of fulcrum and leverage of the mechanics of the body motion.

5. The sore spot in the tendon is the gas block through which the prana cannot flow. Moving this exact spot is the secret of acupuncture. Prana is the medium of acupuncture. It is a force in nature by which anaesthesia can be produced by blocking it or removing the gas block pain factor where it was trapped, locally or generally. That is why this type of anaesthesia does not interfere with consciousness - the patient can talk and eat or drink while under it.

6. That is the great advantage over the chloroform or chemical anaesthesia which drives out the astral body of feeling and consciousness, by producing a molecular change in the bloodstream relationship of the life factor and the oxygen in the red blood cells.

That is why it is so disturbing to the returning astral body or soul - and so dangerous to life. An overdose is fatal. The gross chemistry of anaesthesia does not blend with the life process of prana but disrupts its natural flow and oxidizing power of cells.

7. The root unit is prana - nature's own vital force in all creatures and matter. It is the preserver and sustainer of life in the body. It is the neuter Chi - or Tchi, the vital force which supports all life function through the digestive process of oxidation, assimilation and elimination etc. and feeds all cells and circuits of the body. It is the nourisher - Vishnu Energy - the Preserver - at the Manipura Chakra the navel and solar plexus radiation with the Yin & Yang on each side - top and bottom / inside and out.

Wheel of Life.

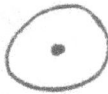

April 10th 1973 Dera. Homeopathy.

The three toxins (miasmas) inherited by genes/*genetics* are psora, syphilis, sychosis (gonorrhoea).

Nature tries to throw *them* out through the skin etc & disease.

Singapore April 28th 1973.

Returned last night from our trip from Kuala Lampur (the Hilton for 3 nights - and sightseeing - and by car to Ipoh 130 miles - where we met a lovely Satsang family with 11 grown up children. Stayed overnight in the Hotel - and drove 103 miles to Penang- and its hills and restaurant on top - and scenery, plus ocean all around. It is an Island and we had rooms in a new Hotel right on the Ocean for 2 nights. Met some good friends of Maharaji who needed help.

We leave here the 30th for Hong Kong. Extract from Yoga in Simple Mudras and Bandhas are more important than asanas and pranayamas for awakening the kundalini shakti, the dormant center of the psychic chakras.

Mudras teach the technique of controlling the involuntary organs.

Bhandas means to tighten or to close. 4 Bhandas are known:

1. Jalandhar B.

2. Uddiyan.

3. Moola B.

4. Maha B.

1. Jalandhar Bhanda- contact throat Muscles and press the chin against the chest. Hold breath.

2. Uddiyan Bhanda — Breathe out fully - contract and draw the stomach muscles in - and upward above the navel portion.

3. Moola Bandha - sit in Padamasana and breathe out, contracting the anus draw it inside.

4. Maha Bandha - sit in Padamasana achieve all 3 at once – hold breath out.

Tratak is meditation - objectivity or extend looking into or at Look steady with eyes wide open. Winkless gazing is called tratak.

Prana means the vitality of life - through organs and breath:

1. in

2. retention.

3. out

Yoga nidra.

Lie flat palms up.

While doing this kriya: don't move any part of your body, and do not sleep.

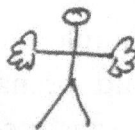

Before starting Yoga nidra make a wish with love and faith - repeat 5 times. Go over the entire body with the attention current - top of the head Sahasrara - (fontanel) the soft spot on a child's head.

forehead chidakash - find darkness everywhere - but behind = light which will appear (mentally). This is all physical. {*Definition CHIDAKASH –that space in front of our closed eyes. When we close our eyes we don't see 'nothing'. We see emptiness. It is the same space that we see when we fall asleep at night and see our dreams. It is like seeing a movie except that the screen is in the mind instead of outside. This screen is called "Chidakash". Chitta-Mind, Akash-Space- Editor*}

In the 4th stage you concentrate on feelings. Feelings of heat or cold - pain or pleasure, hunger or thirst etc.

You can experience any type of feeling without making any type of contact with the object through the process of auto-suggestion and intense imagination.

Feelings are actually experience through imagination - which we may have experienced in the past.

It requires training to change to opposite and hold them. Charma = conceptual concentration on psychic symbol, chakra. The mind becomes very receptive in yoga nidra and is greatly influenced by any firm thought. A strong resolve will penetrate into the deeper layers of consciousness and become potential as it manifests itself in the form of activity on the physical plane.

Shetali pranayama - cooling for high blood pressure, fever and thirst.

Placing the hands on the knees with tongue extended outside and folded. Inhale forcibly through the extended tongue as though trying to swallow the air into the stomach. Practice a short retention breath in Jalandha banda. Exhale slowly through the nose after releasing the bandha and raising the head. This pranayama purifies the blood - prevents and relieves high blood pressure.

Bhastrika pranayama - means bellows.

for asthma – Tuberculosis - pleurisy - gases - phlegm and consumption, for throat and gastric fire.

Plavini pranayama

For hysteria - indigestion and bowel treatment.

Sit in asana - drink in air as drink in water - until the stomach is filled with air. Then pass out the air through the mouth immediately. This cures bowel trouble. Pranic force of life force circulates in the body through the oxygen media, it conducts it.

A man who has mastered his emotion can never get ill unless it is time to leave his mortal abode.

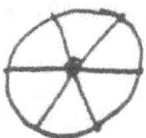

Meditation for a few minutes relieves.

Unite the forces to their Source Center of Balance.

Santa Ana, May 22nd, 1973.

Henri - Cranial Treatment - artery or vein expanded over one side of the head. Treated the outside of the ankle on the heel as the lowest [-] resistance block for that. It brings up the gases locked there - keep at that spot until relieved.

It is a fundamental treatment. The inside under the ankle is for the center of the head - and kidney balance.

For constipation - a simple quick remedy. In 2 cups of hot black coffee, put 2 big tablespoonfuls of <u>cold first pressed</u> unheated olive oil - or sesame oil and drink it. Follow it with hot water and lemon juice - 1 or 2 cups.

Treatment of hip full of gas in the muscles. Patient on the stomach with a pillow or two under the hips, lift up the leg - and work the hips, from the arch, with bending it upward toward the sacrum and rock it in rhythm with it on that side to free the primary respiration cycle.

Put pressure on the ilium articulation downward and toward the center of the spine to relieve the gas pains in it.

Santa Ana, May 24th 1973.

Pierre's Citizen day here.

<u>Treatment for pain in the right hip of Louise</u> last night was most successful. *She was* face down with a pillow or 2 under the hips and I *applied* heavy pressure applied over the right hip - toward the floor and toward the middle line ↑ for sacral articulation.

Also in rhythmic stretches with the sacrum and the leg by flexion.

Excellent results reported this morning – she was free of pain.

June 3rd. Santa Ana, Cal. 4 pm

<u>Heaven:</u> Heaven is but the vision of fulfilled desire.

And hell the shadow from a soul on fire. (Omar Khayyam)

<u>Heart.</u> The heart is the best logician. (Wendell Phillips)

A true heart is better than Gold. (Hanna) ★

A loving heart is the truest Wisdom. (Dickens)

The heart has reasons that reason does not understand. (Boussel)

The ways of the heart, like the ways of providence are mysterious. (Henry Ware)

When the heart speaks, glory itself is an illusion. (Napoleon)

★

Husbands are awkward things to deal with; even keeping them in hot

water will not make them tender. (Mary Buckley)

Marriage is the real cure for love's intoxication. (Helen Rowland)

Never marry but for love; ★

but see what thou lovest is lovely. (Penn)

In Manners, tranquility is the supreme power. (Madame de Maintenon)

Humble wedlock is far better than proud virginity. (Augustine)

Kindness is the golden chain by which society is bound together. (Goethe)

Royalty consists not in vain pomp, but in great virtues. (Agesilaus).

June 18th. 1973 Santa Ana.

1. Treatment to Louise on 17th *in the* evening. She was very low and tired, after a trip to cherry picking and see the Loomis; Lorna, *and* Linda *in* hospital on the way. Nothing had worked - but *she was in* exhaustion. So I started gentle like on the toes - they gave.... but the bottom of the arch was very sore - like the middle of the back and hips. I left the foot on the bed to work with more gentle contacts on the sole and ankle sides, pulling the heel down.

2. She let go - so I could work *more going* deeper and *for* longer. Then I could crack the toes again in the 1st and 2nd joints which gave easily, and continued working on the arch soreness which was still the key. After about 1 hr. she could relax; before all the inside was just a tumble of gas and pain and tension. She hadn't slept at all and so this was a welcome relief. She slept - and was a different person this morning. She was able to take the laundry and bring it back in the hot sun about 11 am. *An 80% improvement.*

3. It is quite clear now - that the 5 elements are the plasma gas matter and the primary bulk of the Universe.

Working with the 5 tattwas is working with the dense primary plasma gas substance and moving the vital current of prana then this electrically charged dense gas - which is the 1st substance of matter in the field of the airy descent of energy into the air element as substance from energy radiation of the repelling electrons - and repelling protons of the atoms of matter.

Conclusion: No matter what the ailment, these 5 currents must flow through matter in 5 circuits for the 5 senses and 5 motor currents to flow to enliven cells and *the* physiology of function.

4. The feet are the negative pole of the body. All the psychic elements are there in a dense precipitation of gas and material and impulsive locks like a crystalline substance of matter. The 5 currents of prana - vital energy must go through to complete its currents of circuits from top to bottom.

The Sound current in the center of the brain and spinal cord also penetrate in the Shushmana current from the Sahansdal Kanwal to the rectum/sacrum.

Nature made an outlet for this subtle gaseous energy in the sole of the feet by placing 2,5000 pores per square inch of skin in the arch of each foot and the hands.

5. So this materialized gas of plasma can flow through the pores as a subtle outlet of the astral light substance in color radiation and as odour from the feet and as perspiration. That explains a lot. Conclusion: When the tension is worked out on the soles of the feet - and the soreness goes - then the currents are flowing naturally again.

Deep yawns means extension of gases - moving in akash – *the* space of matter for relaxation to less dense areas of resistance.

The vital force of prana must reach every cell of matter through subtle etheric currents as in the atom.

6. By experience this becomes an assured procedure to follow:

<u>Not new ways - but deeper stays</u> – More understanding
and concentrated attention can succeed where
everything had failed before.

Even our own short lived effort of the correct technique, when
the patient objected. Even acupuncture needles hurt when
twiddled.

<u>Rule:</u> The patient must understand this process and co-operate,
or it can't be done.

It takes courage and combined effort and mental agreement to
loosen those negative mind patterns of bad habits of thinking
and sensory indulgences. The patient must endure a little pain,
to free the impounded hurts of emotions through crying - or
squirming - or yelling when it hurts. That is natural explosion.

And the doctor must take time to loosen these locks as gently
as can be done - and work twice as long and charge twice as
much. This is a special procedure: not a routine treatment and
that effort and special time must not be taken lightly or
cheapened. It works best when it is appreciated by the patient
in cooperative understanding. Then the impossible is possible.
Do it !

Santa Ana July 1st 1973.

<u>For warts and moles -</u> apply castor oil mixed with white
(decolourised) iodine to them, several times a day. Apply with
small brush in the bottle.

Or massage the castor oil in several times a day - and apply 1
drop of white iodine on them daily.

<u>Breaking finger nail</u> - and peeling ones. Nails are made of protein - use more in the diet.

Bone meal tablets help, also use castor oil & white iodine 1/2 & 1/2 mixed together on them

<u>Split nails lengthwise</u> is a lack of calcium in the system.

Leg cramps are due to a lack of Calcium to balance the phosphorus intake.

Dolomite good or bad? - bad combination of Magnesium & Calcium. Magnesium is anti acid - while Calcium needs acid to digest it.

Vitamin C. has been used to supply the necessary acid for Calcium metabolism.

Calcium - can be Calcium lactate – Calcium gluconate, and bone meal. Bone meal contains phosphorus but the Calcium in it should compensate.

Dolomite is a crushed stone - can lodge in pockets and create trouble although water flowing over it was Dolomite limestone, and was beneficial, as hard water.

In communities of soft water *there are* more heart attacks.

Protective measures for <u>Radium outfall.</u>

In Russia they used sunflower seed as a source of pectin, to attract, bind and eliminate radiation from the system. In Germany buckwheat and millet seeds (or grains) are considered radiation prevention, also sprouts. Alfalfa - soya bean sprouts - etc *you should* get untreated seeds for this.

Creation Theory = all nutrients were present billions of years before science began determining the many nutrients in food. Albert Einstein's Theory of Conservation of Mass Energy confirms the above. Lavoisier's 18th century Theory of Conservation of Matter and Mayer's 19th century, similar Conservation of Energy Theory, "all Matter and Energy can be neither created nor destroyed, but merely changed from one to another" Mass into energy - energy into mass. "What was there is here."

July 14, 1973 70 years in U.S.A.

Elaborate the 5 elements — with the fingers - earth - sweet, smell etc.

5 senses - 5 vices, 5 virtues.

Emotions - Omar Khayyam's quote = desire.

Law of circuits 3 gunas, Sound source & return.

In muscle sprain - work it out, it won't adjust. Louise's pot lifting.

Outlets flow of vital energy-

Astral light currents of space.

Structural impacts through tendons on motion & joints — tension spasm - gas - plasma - in the circuit lines like bubbles.

Sweeping passes to line up magnetic fields and atoms in parallel.

July 19th 3 am 1973

The gunas action, 1. Fire – 3. Air – 2. Water-3.   Sulphur – Mercury - Salt.

The sacred flame - through the eyes united in 3rd eye spirit.

Mornings. Clean palms with Boraxo - rub arch - then massage

with thumbs as the Universal plant life application through absorption.

Clean hands and pure heart = single eye ◉

light to the feet = the way - the truth - the life.

The vital energy current is the Sacred Flame of life - that comes out of the bosom of the earthy nature - the Abel - the younger brother - the animal nature = nature in all living matter. △

The secret Stone of the Philosopher's, crystallized as the One Virtue or power of understanding.

Santa Ana - July 19th 3.20 am 1973

The Subtle Energy Currents applied to the body avenues & outlets in trinity – Superior, Middle & Inferior. Crown, Stem, and roots. *The* Polarity Principle in all Nature.

Do Subtle Energy Polarity 1st *and* then gross application through fluids to reach all cells — to live and thrive in expansion and contraction. Flush the inner fluidic waterways of the brain and spinal cord. Subtle Energy - fluids in the mornings to unite the Currents of life's Ocean. A simple and efficient polarity application in thought & deed. Devotion to the Father of All, the Giver, the Creator, Unity.

Nature's Secret Therapy Rivers:

Breathing pores of the subtle life stream. 2,500, in the palms and arches, *per square inch*. Only 400 per square inch in the skin.

The fire of the eyes - the power of the thighs and dancing feet.

The skill and touch of the hands - the dancing feet - root support of Nature.

Superior 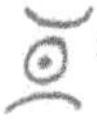 Nature = Consciousness in all.

The Conqueror of Nature "Christos - the spirit incarnate", who overcame all - the Christ, the hope of glory in us — in the bosom of the Infinite always.

July 20th Santa Ana 6am 1973.

Structure is the Elemental Gas of plasma with its 5 sensory and motor provision for Soul function and awareness of Inner Realization of Energy glow from the Soul and the Cosmos.

Structure is form — crystallized plasmic function is life = soul energy and cosmic energy of nature flowing through the form.

Soul is consciousness, the eternal Bhagavan taking form in matter as the Shabda incarnate - Shabda is the Holy Spirit or Eternal Sound Current. The Father is the Creator = Radha Soami Himself the Unknown & Unconditioned.

July 20th 1973 Santa Ana.

I gave Louise a treatment - time 1 hr. – *she was* relieved after a month of pain.

The puzzle of hip pains over the buttocks - that nothing would relieve.

The patient wanted to pound the buttocks and hips.

An indigestion symptom of gases lodged there and in the thigh with great pain especially at night. *The* Fire principle *was* locked up as gases.

The puzzle was solved by polarity locally applied. Heavy steady pressure over the painful thigh - then I *worked* the leg tendons and calf of the leg *releasing* the sore locks I found and traced along tendons, then the foot - on the cuboid articulation edge - and the transverse arch top and bottom - held firm while working the upper leg areas.

July 20th 10.30 pm.

The Treatment to Louise *was* a real discovery of advanced work of *the* coordination of 1. Superior. 2. Middle & 3. Inferior regions.

Superior. Shoulders from the back. A very sensitive contact under the tip of the shoulder - pushing it up with the elbow to get under it, for a lifting severe hold - it is a real Acupuncture point of the airy triad region motor function.

It effects the prana in the throat and airy locks in *the* Anterior 1st. & 2nd *cervical* area. (*possibly dorsal rather cervical implied here. Editor*)

Combined with the elbow lift and push upward - and pressure on the hip with the right elbow - supporting all with the head in a four point contact simultaneously. A New *technique*. The Patient is lying on the side with the operator sitting on a stool in the back using both hands elbows and head in the upper triad locks and the trunk including the hips.

The low triad - from the hips down go with the feet acupuncture points, like the cuboid soreness around the edges - goes with the anterior & lateral thigh soreness of digestion reflex and the lateral side of the outer ankle.

It all reveals itself as you work. One flows out and into the next regional approach superior & inferior Polarity, lateral and anterior or posterior regions on back, shoulders and hips.

It is a simple miracle approach - from the back - with the patient on the side and the operator sitting on a stool in the back of the patient linking top and bottom posteriorly and laterally, with vital reflexes or acupuncture points without a puncture. Just finding and moving blocks.

The shoulder tip is the most vital and sore point. The buttocks soreness and legs can be released by the triad procedure of each section - thigh and upper leg - calf - and foot, relating each to the other by deep compression and following the tendon soreness.

The etheric energy is a subtle fluid. The physical energy is a gross fluid both must flow and blend to nourish tissue cells

The violin is like the body.

The strings of the violin and the connective tissue must vibrate to the Sound Current impact – as the+/- motivating factor.

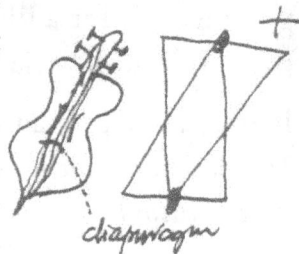

diaphragm

The 2,500 pores per square inch in the palm of the hand are outlets like a sieve - for the fine Astral Light Energy of the Vital Current of the 1,000 Petalled Lotus in Sahansdal Kanwal region which animates the Universe and creatures.

There are 3 special radiant outlets *in the skull plus* 2 currents from the eyes expressing the brain *function*,

2 currents from the palms of the hands and 2 currents from the arch of the feet express motion, the vital spring in the step or dancing feet.

Vibrant motion is in the strings as expression of Energy.

The pores and hollow organs are for the neuter airy & gaseous energy for secretion and digestion which *consists* of assimilation, elimination & oxidation - to supply the materials for cellular replacement of worn out cells and *to give* nourishment to all cells – physiological function.

The Tendon collagen fibres convey lymph and cerebrospinal fluid through the tendons and ligaments - animating the frame as motion by fulcrum (articulation & flexion) and leverage through muscle function.

July 24th 1973 Santa Ana.

That steady gas pain in the hips and thighs can be relieved by finding the block in each section along the bones - the thigh, the knee - the ankle and the foot. Also by firm deep compression of the muscles - alternately as Polarity [+] and [-]. It is an anaemia and digestive symptom made worse by taking too much blood from the patient for analysis - (*In* Louise's case: 24, 1 oz vials, over *a* 1 month time *period*).

Emotions can produce any symptom or pain complaint. From angina to throat pressure and exhaustion - fainting symptoms and gas no end.

July 25th. 1973 Santa Ana.

When tendons and arches of the feet, are released and are not too sore anymore then the physical condition is good, regardless what the patient complains of. Emotions can cause real pain symptoms and pressure in the head, *disturb* the solar plexus energy flow and *create* gas pains in the spine itself. They reoccur

121

when relieved, because the real cause is not removed. A lot of scientific checks with instruments and x-rays and blood tests are more convincing than all suggestion or other proof. The emotion is the real psychology involved.

July 25th. 1973 Santa Ana. ★

HCl Therapy. Gas and indigestion is more often caused by a lack of hydrochloric acid - to digest even the iron when given as well as the food, it is not hyperacidity but fermentation due to indigestion caused by a lack of HCl present in *the stomach*.

Dr Tucker, after trying many types, prescribed tablets of hydrochloric acid - betaine with pepsin with great success. HCl digests the protein. Apple cider vinegar and water given before meals - is less effective. But it increases the haemoglobin in the blood when given to animals - proved by later autopsy.

B12 is a must - for vegetarians – when using this HCl supplementation.

August 3rd 1973 Santa Ana.

1 tablespoonful of seawater taken daily or whole sea salt - for arthritis (in a deficiency disease) given on their cereal. April - Let's Live magazine 1973. Then spryness in walking over all others. (*Presumably a reference the difference between the group using salt and to a control group not taking it. Editor*)

Natural oils have lecithin in them.

Aug. 3rd 1973 Santa Ana. California.

Millet is the only cereal with an alkaline reaction and is an excellent food for diabetics.

Aug. 4th 1973 Santa Ana.

Mount Meru – *Mount* Sumeru & Kailash

Mount Sinai – *Mount* Horeb & Arrarat.

Sore muscles are gas pockets in them – use pressure - solid pressure on restless twitching legs, and thighs and ankles and arches. (Louise)

Aug. 5th 1973. Santa Ana.

Honey is recommended for fertility by Dr. Frances Seymour of N.Y.

2 tablespoonfuls of honey after breakfast and 2 tablespoonfuls of honey at bed time. She (*Dr Seymour*) said it worked.

A mixed variety of honey — dark and light - substitute for cane sugar.

Constipation & Anaemia overcome as causes.

Leonardo da Vinci, in the 15 century, used the principle of the four polarized elements of earth, air, fire and water for all his scientific discoveries which anticipated most of our modern inventions. The soundness of this foundation and its adaptability for its future discoveries implies and open challenge to the science of our age.

Aug. 5th 1973.

Einstein and Relativity, from the Ambala Tribune, March 16th, 1958. (A cut-out article on file).

On foods in India: are either Thanda cooling or Garam - heating on the system.

Luther Burbank once said: "If mankind would seriously devote itself to its own physical regeneration, the human race would not only be freed from all disease, but most forms of crime would be eliminated."

Aug. 5th 1973.

Life is a feeling - throbbing sensory and motor organic motivation in tissue form of cells as a living unit - or composition of cellular groups in organic growing bodies to experience Life in form, as human, animal - vegetable with enzymatic action as its unit background.

Enzymes are easily destroyed by heat - or boiling point of 100C. 40C is their average function thermal in organisms to promote reactions in animals and plants. They are slow in reactions and can be used up completely.

Proteins are the usual carriers also the cerebro-spinal fluid - formed in the brain as the life fluid carrier.

Catalysts are mostly metals -> platinum, copper, silver, nickel and activated charcoal.

In non-metallic elements, salts and more complex compounds are all found among catalysts employed at the present time; the active agent is most frequently a specific metal, or metallic oxide. Catalysts are not thermo-labile - inorganic - function at

1OOC to 5OOC of heat. They act by mere presence and are not used up - (like organic enzymes). Facilitate action in industrial operation - (like plating metals) Platinum must be present for plating metals.

3. Enzymes = Biological matter impregnated with vital energy values.

Aug. 6th 1973.

Treatment to Louise.

1.Sitting up sideways on a chair is the best position for a real head drain - for eyes, ears, neck, atlas, occiput, etc. and reaching down with the heel of the hand while tilting the head way back with a real fulcrum on the upper dorsals, including the 2nd - 3rd – 4th – 5th - 6th or even the 7th & 8th when they are congested.

Then have the patient lean forward and put the elbows across the knees, allows the spine to spring and give freely without support

2. Better than on a table you can open up all the upper dorsals over the spinous processes and the transverse as well as over the ribs and articulations, by merely turning the hands to fit over the ribs as support.

Then lift the shoulder especially on the tense side [-] [+] (head symptom side) slip the hand under the lower shoulder tip, lift it up on your knee support and make your knuckles get a good contact on the ribs and articulations with pressure forward and upward lifting - under the blade as well as all around it. It does wonders - for neck & head & ribs & dorsals.

3. Chiropractic 1st aid book $5. (*written by Dr Stone's friend and colleague Major De Jarnette. Editor*) For throbbing pains - light pressure on 3rd & 4th dorsal constricts the blood vesselsof the brain, when it is hyperemic. Heavy pressure dilates the blood vessels in the brain in case of fevers - this gives definite relief. In the case of anaemic headaches, this pressure is invaluable and gives definite relief.

Dorsal *vertebrae* 3 *and* 4 control the eyes as constrictors. Pain in the eyes is due to dilation and its resultant effect. Pressure is quickly relieved by light pressure on 3rd, 4th Dorsals

Iritis is a good example where this helps.

Pressure of a light nature at the 3rd, 4th, 5th Dorsal constricts the blood vessels in the ear. While pressure on the 7th exit of the cranial nerve dilates these vessels. The 7th cranial nerve area is directly anterior to the meatus of the ear, A distance of 1½ inches, it dilates.

4. To constrict the membranes of the nose, apply light pressure to 2nd, 4th and 5th Dorsal. *In* nasal congestion this will help greatly. To dilate these membranes make pressure on the 7th cranial area. Pressure on the zygomatic process will often times cause the stomach to discharge its contents and prove helpful in treating cases that are unable to turn in bed. Pressure here, quickly relieves gas pains.

5. Pressure on the upper lip controls the spleen and pancreas. Use in diabetes. Chin tip, effects colon = evacuation, and stimulates the rectum.

Prostate gland is effected by pressure under the chin - for under-activity. Pressure applied to top of the head is most useful in controlling nervous conditions.

To stimulate lungs make pressure from 4th to 8th Dorsal.

To dilate blood vessels of the eye make pressure on the 5th cranial nerve at its exit - 2" inferior to the eye near the articulations of the nose. Dorsal 3, 4, 5 control the eyes as constrictors and ears. (For Iritis). Pain in the eye is due to dilation.

6. (Casey) Pressure on the 3rd cervical relaxes the whole body. Its the neutral middle.

10th & 11th Dorsal to Peyers Gland = the origin of poison in sciatica and rheumatism. Charcoal tablets also heavy salt packs, hot to perspire.

Camphorated oil on scars. Sinusitis 9th Dorsal down. Stuttering = 3rd cervical, 2nd & 3rd Dorsal. 2nd, 3rd & 5th cervical.

Mullein tea for varicose veins – *steep until cool.*

Warm castor oil packs for felons (*a purulent inflammation of the end joint of a finger, sometimes affecting the bone. Sometimes called a whitlow Editor*) - also good for neck and stiff joints.

Rub castor oil into the scalp and massage it deeply.

For stomach ulcers use hot castor oil packs - appendicitis - gall bladder. colitis - and <u>for obstructions </u>in intestines - cured overnight.

Also use it for high blood pressure and for abscessed and painful joints or fingers.

7. For kidneys and balance between the pancreas and bladder use the Jerusalem artichoke - cook them in Parchment paper - to hold all *the medicinal* values.

For dropsy - use watermelon seed tea – ½ cup of crushed seeds in a quart of water - steep for ½ hour. - Drink a glass a day for 3 to 4 days then repeat.

For sore feet and swollen ankles - rub the lumbar area with olive oil and myrrh. It's caused by acidity. Use hot and cold applications. Also camphorated oil soda - for very painful feet, bathe in solution of Soda water - a saturated solution as hot as possible for 2O min every other day.

8. Witch hazel for feet toes and itch. *To add* Luster *to* hair and increase it's growth use cooked Irish potato peeling - in Patar *parchment* paper to hold values.

For bad breath use Glycothymoline (*an Edgar Cayce remedy, Editor*) - 5-6 drops in drinking water.

Coca Cola syrup - 1 oz in plain water as a drink helps kidney and bladder *function*.

For moles - warts, cysts use castor oil or touch up with 200/10 (5%) solution of hydrochloric acid.

Diabetes - massage with peanut oil only over the small of the back, sacrum and hips.

For sore tired feet and stiff joints - bathe them in old hot coffee grounds, and rub the bursa and limbs well - the acid will aid in eliminating all heaviness in throat and chest.

9. For high blood pressure - the power of peanut oil and camphorated oil helps.

Light spinal massage - no heavy treatment

Castor oil packs for abdominal obstructions and swollen feet. It stimulates the lymphatic tissue and organs.

Use 8" flannel - 3 thicknesses - apply hot – 1½ to 3 hrs keep it warm with a lamp. It stimulates the defence mechanisms. & lymph production. Miracles follow. Take olive oil and lemon after it for 3 days. Also used in chronic ulcerated colitis, due to trauma & shock. Also used for kidney stones and in all lymph stasis - cancer - psoriasis - arthritis - on moles and warts, cysts - gout.

For knots around the joints of fingers use Epsom salts - applied.

10. Salt packs for improved circulation. Alium sativa (garlic) used in Tibet for chest and asthma.

Cayce's business advice - Listen to the still small voice - not outside!

Colds are due to over acidity, keep *your body* alkaline.

All yellow foods have Vitamin B. Green light is healing.

Cabbage for pin worms = use greens - cause is milk.

Asthma - 9th Dorsal. Take l to 5 grains of calcidine in water for relief.

(*Calcidine was an old fashioned remedy, sometimes recommended by Edgar Cayce, and was a tablet which, when dissolved in water was indicated for dry cough and scant secretions. It was a compound containing iodide of lime, a 15% available iodine in combination with lime and starch. It was mostly produced by Abbott Laboratories and was generally available from the mid 1930s onwards. Possibly superseded by the Cayce remedy "atomidine." Editor*)

For Baldness massage the scalp with crude oil, then white Vaseline once of week. Iodine deficiency - acts upon skin, nails and hair.

11. 3rd cervical & 3rd & 4th lumbar - act on the thyroid - use sea food - kelp - carrots - onions & garlic.

Blood poison - use salt and turpentine to saturate around it - not on it, then use hot packs on it

In lock jaw and infections - hot packs of it over the legs 3 / 4 times daily - fruit juice diet. Tannic acid, the Ungantine (*possibly turpentine. Editor*) or oil.

For scars use Ungantine or camphorated oil - cutting off the air relieves pain.

"Healing through attitude" - "I am sick and going to stay sick" ? Attitude toward others, how long ? *To hold* a grudge -

12. Haemorrhoids - rising on toes contract rectum upward - udan lift (Uddiyana Bandha), cat stretch. Bleeding piles - Pazo Ointment. (*an old remedy from the Paris Medicine Co., St. Louis, Mo. It is no longer available editor*) No spices or carbonated drinks - cold water and lemon.

Love grows on Love - Love gives,
Love forgiveth - Love endures,
Love understands, Love is opportunity for overcoming hardships, and ego.
Life is living "Thy will be done". Discipline.

Continuous constructive effort is essential. Ask yourself – Lord what should I do? Life is what we put into it.

Granulated eyelids - use 2 oz. Boric Acid - or a scraped Irish potato over the eye, then wash the eye with glycothymoline.

13. Cayce. Castor Oil packs for breaking up adhesions - appendicitis and impactions.

Granulated eyelids - use 2oz boric acid - solution is tops (*?editor*)+ 10% myrrh tincture. Eyes - 2nd cervical. 7th-9th Dorsal. Treat with soda in salt solution in water - 3 to 1.

Diet.

Add lime or lemon juice to 1 to 4 orange juice. Acid foods = all combination of fats and sugars and starches are acid forming. 20% acid - 80% alkaline goods. Never take pickles which produce acids in the lower part of the stomach. Vinegar etc acetic acid. In Tuberculosis. the kidneys go bad first. Meats should be taken with things below the ground like potatoes - skin is best.

14. Don't mix onions, radishes with celery or lettuce at the same time. *Having them* Separate *is* OK. Just before meals take mild saffron (*original text looked like safran*. Editor)tea; it coats the whole stomach.

Sugar sours the stomach; add lime or lemon juice to orange and grapefruit juice.

Use 3 vegetables above the ground to 1 below. Lemon & lime juice are good alkalinizers.

Drink mullein tea fresh daily.

Gelatine salads act as a catalyst to the digestion & absorption of vitamins. Grate vegetables fine and add to the gelatine.

Calcium foods are carrots, lettuce leaf and potato skins etc.

Citrus fruits - natural warm milk.

Iron foods are raisins, grapes, lentil, red cabbage, berries, pears.

15. Onions, asparagus, vitamin A for brain, bones and nerves.

Vitamin B6 & B (*?editor*) for energy of the nerve force and tendons.

Vitamin C for face and tendinous muscles of the jaw.

G(*editor*) for the sympathetic system.

Vitamins A & D are not stored in the body. Use citrus fruits daily.

B. (*?Editor*)gives calcium, silicon & iron.

Creaking sound in neck = un (*possibly occipital as occ. editor?*) balance with 3rd Cervical. Deafness - 5th 6th Dorsal vertebrae.

Castor oil packs over the liver and gall ducts for 1½ hours twice a day, for 3 days each week.

Then take olive oil - in teaspoonful doses - 3 - 4 times a day.

Sterate of zinc as powder with Balsam of Johnson & Johnson can be applied to the skin.

16. Cleansing diet - 3 days on raw apples - the olive oil.

Diabetes = the Jerusalem artichoke raw - then cooked - alternately. It has insulin; use leafy vegetables & honey. Artichokes keep best in the ground or flowerpot. Can be obtained from seeds - Burgess Seed & Plant Co., Galesburg, Mich. or Walker Robinson Farm, Home, Penns. 1 almond a day - keeps the Dr. away. No carbonated drinks. Sometimes just carbonated water is recommended in hot weather for lymph stasis.

Tea is more harmful than plain coffee – *coffee is* without tannin. No milk with either - (bad.)

17. Formulas; Poison neutralizers & gargle, apple cider vinegar, 1 teaspoonfuls to a 6 oz glass of water, if the finger nails bent back or tear easily or split - use 1 teaspoonful of cider vinegar *with* each meal.

For reducing ...

1 tsp. of cider vinegar in a glass of water, sip during meal.

Fingernails - longitudinal ridges means thyroid - thick and slow growth, deficiency. Smooth & hyperflexible = Anterior pituitary.

Ca Phos – *vitamin* B 2 - g. (*? Editor*) & protein.

Aug .10th Santa Ana 7 pm.

Louise went to meet Maxine (*Pierre Pannetier's wife. Editor*) to go to the airport for Dorothy from Miami

Aug. 10th Santa Ana 1973.

The psoas magnus muscle treatment. Relaxation on the table and the primitive Indian squatting posture to keep it pliable and useful naturally.

Show the tablework - the mechanics & technique - and the squat the easy way -

and rock on the ankle joint for stretching.

The treatment for the lower half of the body - sitting up treatment for the upper half.

Simple correction for occipital spinal muscle tension. Have 2 pillows and a little one on top - to fit under the occiput. Lie on the back with a roll or pillow under the knees to relax the leg. It is a most restful posture, for thinking - or day dreaming relaxation for all spinal & neck muscles and psoas muscles.

Santa Ana, August 13th 1973.

Notes; The Pubococcygeus muscle has 4th & 5th sacral nerve supply. Part of levator ani muscle. The Iliococcygeus group muscles. Pouparts Ligament. Rectal contraction - lifting up these muscles for tone and power.

The four Vital <u>Emotional Temperaments</u>

1. Sanguine = air = Oneiromancy dream divination

2. The Bilious (*choleric. Editor*) = fire = pyromancy & magnetism

3. The Phlegmatic = water = to hydromancy by crystal ball

4. The Melancholic = earth = geomancy and cartomancy.

1 Sanguine disposition is a naturally cheerful, hopeful, confident - ruddy faced, blood red complexion, red iron oxide crayons.

2 The Bilious temperament - (fire) peevish, petty, cross - testy - physical pathology of excess bile - liver treatment.

After the energy currents are set in motion, then it takes lots of liquids to flush out the sedimentations in all cells = it's a laundry process all the way through physiologically. Don't depend on the good polarity treatment alone - that is the power current through the tattwas - mental - emotional - physical.

Mind plane - 1 Thought direction

Vital plane - 2. Feeling - attention

Physical plane - 3 Body structures

Aug. 13th. 1973.

Every thought changes the valence and polarity of the astral body. (the Vital Emotions) Will is concentrated thought which controls the astral body and surcharges it and environment.

Paracelsus. Born Nov. 11th 1493 - 48 year old died Sept. 24th - 1541.

Archeus = Lebenscraft - Vital Energy - Prana.

Sant Ana, Aug 14th 1973.

A resume of a high protein diet for vegetarians - who believe in a big breakfast.

Breakfast.

6 - 8 oz of skim milk powder.

1 heaping teaspoonful of soybean powder.

6 teaspoonful sunflower seeds - (blended)

2 Bananas

1 teaspoonful - Brewers Yeast - soybean lecithin and wheat germ.

Spring water.

Lunch.

1 garlic clove

1 oz bunch of parsley = (for chlorophyll to counteract the odour, and for vitamin and mineral content)

1 carrot

4 red lettuce leaves - unfiltered apple juice.

Dinner

1 protein - 1 cooked veg & fresh fruit.

Santa Ana - Aug. 14th 1973.

A real polarity treatment to Dorothy - with a shoulder & neck pain for 7 years - after a whiplash injury.

Lots of treatments from M.Ds - chiropractors and masseurs. The sitting-up special polarity treatment did it. The upper ribs on the right side were too high (and turned bottom edge up). Treatment . The elbow arm lift 1st on the right shoulder. Then muscle spasm release over the shoulders - and under them then as a lift - it gave beautifully at 2nd and 3rd Dorsal spine. It was locked there anteriorly.

The right shoulder raised up at once.

There also was a lumbar muscle lock released.

Santa Ana - Aug. 27th 1973.

We had a most successful Polarity Convention here a finished yesterday.

1. Some outstanding findings in Polarity Therapy were - The Positive pole contractions in the occipital bone attachment of the ascending central tendon of the erector spinal muscles on either side as a motor tension block.

It is equally as important as the sensory 10th cranial tension in front of the neck = the pneumo-gastric parasympathetic nerve. Emily and two cases from Havana - and one from San Francisco were good proof.

2. Working with these 2 occiput tension blocks - seems the answer to many deep neck and motor contraction pains and it is surprising how resistant they are - it takes more time to work them out than we had previously given them - that is why they were overlooked: The Anterior 10th and these 2 make up [-] the [+] balance & the 11 parasympathetic digestive motor nerve tract and its contact. It was a most rewarding to find in Emily and several specially hard cases to solve. And it did it all.

Aug. 28th Santa Ana.

Pain in the calf of the legs is gas - due to rich and too much food.

Use herb teas and orange juice for a few days.

Eye pain - can be relieved from the occiput by reaching over the head and pulling forward - contact at the motor center - near the middle of the occiput on that sore & tight tendon there. It is a major obstruction and lesion. - A definite find - a block of great importance - in the occiput + motor area. A real active meridian + lock for all motor lesions below - even in the thigh and abdomen. Anterior = a motor spasm control.

Aug 30th 1973

Iblis refused to bow before Adam when all the angels were brought before him and Il (*incomprehensible writing. Editor*) and Lib (to name them) bowed to him.

Urea is a chemical combination of carbon dioxide and ammonia. Dissolved in water it reduced the conductivity for electrical currents, by polymerization of other salts, into less ionized forms, for urea is known to promote the colloidal state

137

of matter (a state essential to life) from the crystalloidal state.

Urea, if present in pericellular fluids, would reduce the conductivity of the cell. It maintains the osmotic balance between semi permeable membranes . Blood normally contains 25 to 50 mg. of urea, per 100cc or about 10% of its sodium chloride content.

When adrenocortin is deficient, salt is lost through the kidneys and blood urea rises, a compensatory effect.

In cortin deficiency it has been shown that the kidney tubules let through more salts and reabsorb more urea.

A fact not commonly known is that urea's a normal plant juice constituent too which would indicate that it is essential to most cell activity.

3. Nutrition: tip of the month: <u>Diverticulosis.</u> Recent tests on rats indicate that diverticulosis (intestinal) can be overcome through the use of bulk forming foods, such as whole wheat products.

A note at the end of the book.

Lex Barker - the Tarzan Man after Weissmuller dropped dead on the street in New York at 53. June paper Betty Grable with the million dollar legs died at 56 - July 3rd 1973.

It is a deeper subtle energy that governs Life and its relation to the World.

Chapter References

Acknowledgments

1. A copy of this copyright permission is available on the website www.pranotherapy.com

Preface

1. http://www.pranotherapy.com is the web site linked to this book. It contains a wealth of extra material relating to the Dewanchand Varma and Dr Randolph Stone.

Introduction

1. The five main original books on Polarity Therapy were in published order; Energy - the Vital Principle in the Healing Arts, The Wireless Anatomy of Man, Polarity Therapy - Its Triune Function, The Mysterious Sacrum and Vitality Balance. The 25 Charts and the Appendix to Wireless Anatomy appeared later. The small pamphlets included, Health Building, Easy Stretching Postures for Health and Vitality, A purifying diet as well as some extra course handouts form the 1970s.

2. Nan was not actually my grandmother but a professional nanny who went into service with my grandmother after the First World War.

3. The Ether of Space by Sir Oliver Lodge. Published by Harper and Brothers, London and New York 1909.

4. Representative texts that Stone would have read were The Chakras by Charles Leadbeater, Occult Chemistry: Investigations by Clairvoyant Magnification into the Structure of the Atoms of the Periodic Table and Some Compounds by Annie Besant and Charles Leadbeater. The Etheric Double and other titles by Arthur E. Powell. All these books were originally published by the Theosophical Publishing House, Wheaton, Illinois, USA and London, England.

The Evolution of Technique

1. Leon Chaitow ND DO and Judith DeLany LMT have written numerous authoritative text books on Neuromuscular Technique.

Modern Neuromuscular Techniques 3rd Edition, Churchill Livingstone ISBN - 978-0443069376

Clinical Application of Neuromuscular Techniques Volume 1: Upper Body 2nd edition, Churchill Livingstone/Elsevier , ISBN - 978-0-443-07448-6

Clinical Application of Neuromuscular Techniques Volume 2: Lower Body 2nd edition, ISBN - 978 - 0443068157

Clinical Application of Neuromuscular Techniques - Practical Case Study Exercises, Churchill Livingstone/Elsevier, ISBN - 978-0-443100000

2. Dr Randolph Stone major books have been collected into three volumes as below

Polarity Therapy The Complete Collected Works Volume 1, Book Publishing Company ISBN - 978-1570670794

Polarity Therapy The Complete Collected Works Volume 2, Book Publishing Company ISBN - 978-1570670800

Health Building - The Conscious Art of Living Well, Book Publishing Company ISBN - 978-1570670817

3. The Dr Randolph Stone virtual Museum is at http:///www.polaritynetwork.com

4. The Dr Randolph Stone lectures 1956 - 1965. A double audio DVD produced by MWI Publishing.

Vitalism

1. Stone referred to this fact in one of his audio lectures where he mentioned that the osteopathic journal refused to take his course adverts. Apparently, Stone had for years regularly sent them articles relating to energetic processes which were clearly not well received.

2. Quantum-Touch: The Power to Heal (Third Edition) by Richard Gordon, North Atlantic Books, ISBN- 978-1556435942

3. Energy Medicine: The Scientific Basis by James L. Oschman, Churchill Livingstone ISBN -978-0443062612

4. The Wine of Life and other essays on Societies, Energy and living things by Harold J. Morowitz, published St Martins Press 1979 USA. Abacus UK 1981.

5. Over the years I have heard this story and subtle variants from numerous Feldenkrais practitioners and teachers, notably Eileen Bach y Rita and Garet Newell.

6. Spiritualism and Occultism by Dion Fortune. Thoth Publications. ISBN - 978-1-870450-38-6

7. Applied Magic and Aspects of Occultism by Dion Fortune. Thoth Publications ISBN - 978-0850306651

8. Tertium Organum and A New Model of the Universe by P. D. Ouspensky. Both of the titles were written between in the early 1900s but the content is extraordinary and still relevant today.

Dewanchand Varma - A Brief Biography

1. Copies of the newspaper articles on these court cases from the French newspapers of the day plus English translations are available on the web site at http://www.pranotherapy.com

2. Copies of these articles and photographs are available on the web site at http://www.pranotherapy.com

3. The UK patent number for the finger exercise device is GB 568609 (A). Full copies of the patents of this an other devices are also available on the web site at http://www.pranotherapy.com

Connective Tissue

1. The original audio of these transcriptions are available on the web site at http://www.pranotherapy.com

2. This meeting may have taken place even earlier as records show Stanley

Lief ND DC travelled to the USA earlier to both study and teach in 1936 and in 1947. In the 1947 trip Lief attended the National Chiropractic Association's Annual convention in July in Omaha where he taught a seminar intriguingly entitled 'New Concepts in Manipulative Techniques.' Its also possible Stone and Lief met more than once. The probable dating of this meeting comes from the fact that Stone gave Lief copies of his books and as Stone's books were not all in print before the late 1950s it sets the later time frame. I am indebted to Leon Chaitow for this information on the books in Stanley Lief's library.

Stone's report of the technique as being painful is curious as this is not majorly born out by Varma's own writings and the fact that the Neuromuscular Technique that evolved from Varma's work is not intrinsically a painful technique though it has been through a long evolution.

3. From 'Clef de la Santé,' translated from the French.

4. Initis – Congestion of the Connective Tissues by Dr Andrea Rabagliati. Pioneers in Manual Therapy Volume II. MWI Publishing. 2012.

Polarity Books from MWI Publishing

POLARITY THERAPY – Healing with Life Energy by Alan Siegel and Phil Young
ISBN: 978-0954445058

THE ART OF POLARITY THERAPY – A Practitioner's Perspective by Phil Young

Pioneers of Manual Therapy Volume II
INITIS –Congestion of the Connective Tissues
by Dr Andrea Rabagliati

For further information on
Polarity
and
Polarity training

www.masterworksinternational.com
www.polaritynetwork.com

The Dr Stone Lectures
1956 -1965
Audio DVD

This is a unique archive containing 12 hours of lecture material by the creator of Polarity Therapy. A must for all serious students of Polarity.

The DVDs cover a series of Dr Stone's lectures given between 1956 and 1965 that have been digitally re-mastered and enhanced.

Available from

www.masterworksinternational.com

www.ingramcontent.com/pod-product-compliance
Lightning Source LLC
Chambersburg PA
CBHW050223270326
41914CB00003BA/543